Invisible Trauma

Invisible Trauma

The Psychosocial Effects of Invisible Environmental Contaminants

Henry M. Vyner, M.D.
Radiation Research Institute

Lexington Books
D.C. Heath and Company/Lexington, Massachusetts/Toronto

Library of Congress Cataloging-in-Publication Data

Vyner, Henry M.
  Invisible trauma.

  Bibliography: p.
  Includes index.
    1. Pollution—Environmental aspects.   2. Pollu-
  tants—Environmental aspects.   3. Pollution—Psycho-
  logical aspects.   I. Title.   II. Title: Psychosocial
  effects of the invisible environmental contaminants.
  [DNLM: 1. Environmental Health.   2. Environmental
  Pollution—adverse effects.   3. Psychophysiologic
  Disorders.   4. Stress, Psychological—etiology.
  WA 670 V996i]
  TD174.V95   1987   363.7'32   85–46019
  ISBN 0–669–12804–X (alk. paper)

Published simultaneously in Canada
Printed in the United States of America
International Standard Book Number: 0–669–12804–X
Library of Congress Catalog Card Number: 85–46019

The paper used in this publication meets the minimum requirements of
American National Standard for Information Sciences—Permanence of
Paper for Printed Library Materials, ANSI Z39.48–1984. ∞™

88 89 90 91 8 7 6 5 4 3 2 1

To
Karinna

Contents

Foreword

In recent years, names such as "Love Canal," "Three Mile Island," "Seveso," and "Chernobyl" have come to represent not only the places where technological disasters have occurred, but also the enormous problems attendant on our attempts to cope with the consequences of the disasters, and to mitigate the effects of like disasters in the future—if we cannot totally prevent their occurrence. At the heart of the coping and mitigation problems lies what Henry Vyner calls "the mystery"; at this late-twentieth-century date, we know little more about the health effects of exposure to radiation, chemical, and other invisible industrial contaminants than fourteenth-century Europeans knew about the cause and prevention of the Plague.

The reasons for our collective ignorance can be pinpointed to the relative newness of the presence of such invisible contaminants in the world, our even more recent awareness of the possibility that they may create adverse effects on living beings and the environment, and the social context that determines and often limits which health problems will be accorded our collective attention and resources. Whatever the complex sets of reasons, the amount of solid information about the effects of invisible industrial contaminants is miniscule, relative to the amount that we need in order to make information-based policy decisions about them, at the individual and collective societal level.

Miniscule as our information is about the effects of invisible contaminants on physical health, we are even less informed about the psychological and social responses to the experience of contamination by invisible agents, and about the interplay of such responses and the development of physical symptoms. As his task, Vyner has undertaken to shed light upon this problem. In *Invisible Trauma*, he draws upon his dual background in medicine and social science to examine every known case study in the English language on the psychosocial effects of invisible contamination, including his own interview-based studies of atomic veterans. His analysis of the case studies, starting with a discussion of the Plague, is rich and interesting in itself. It is important that the author draws generalizations, because many reports of the health, social, and psychological effects of technological disasters have been criticized as "anecdotal," "only one case," and "having no comparison group." He used the generalizations in two important ways. First, he used them to enrich and alter existing paradigms about human coping and stress and to add to the emerging theories about traumatic neurosis or posttraumatic stress disorder. Second, he used them to examine the effects of institutional denial on the psychological and physical responses of people exposed to invisible environmental contaminants. Vyner concludes that when government agencies, physicians, industries, and others who should be concerned deny that the victims are suffering at all, blame them for their symptoms, or refuse them the help and the sympathy that they need, then they exacerbate the problems created by invisible contaminants. He links policy recommendations for the provision of help with the theoretical stance he has developed, based on the evidence he has examined.

This work then is a solid contribution in an area where there is a great need for scholarly work, tempered by a sensible approach that takes into account the social context of problem development and attempts at problem solution.

Adeline Gordon Levine
Sociology Department
SUNY/Buffalo

1
Introduction

A brief inspection of the history of industrialization reveals that the industrial age has truly transformed our lives on this planet. Surely, this transformation has been a mixed blessing. The fruits of our industrial labor are the commodities that it has made available to the people of the world: steel, automobiles, televisions, synthetic fibers and substances, and a cornucopia of electrical appliances. Industrialization has also created massive amounts of capital, material wealth, and a higher standard of living for many who live in the industrialized societies.

In tandem with this material prosperity, industrialization has also given us increased population densities, the disruption of ecological systems, the disappearance of wilderness and agricultural land, and the contamination of the environment in which we live.

Until recently, the threat of environmental contamination has been understood solely in terms of its biological effects. Scientists have more than begun the important task of making us aware of the deleterious biological effects that environmental contaminants have had on plant and animal life. In contrast, only during the past decade have we become more than intuitively aware of the psychosocial effects of environmental contamination. The scientific investigation of these psychosocial effects has been more or less forced upon us by several major accidents involving invisible environmental contaminants. The exposures that occurred at Three Mile Island and at Love Canal probably played the largest role in introducing society to this problem.

This book looks at all of the existing studies published in the English language on the psychosocial effects of the invisible environmental contaminants. Since this is a new field, only a limited amount of studies have been done to date on this problem. Nonetheless, within this small body of research one finds striking parallels between findings of the existing case studies. A central task of this book is to point out and delineate these parallel findings in order to: (1) describe the principal psychosocial effects of exposure to the invisible environmental contaminants, (2) stimulate further research in this area by pointing out the many unanswered questions in the field, and (3) provide some early knowledge on the basis of which public policy and medical care issues can be defined and discussed.

In this comparative case study approach, *Invisible Trauma* draws principally on studies of the psychosocial effects of the invisible contaminants as they have been found at the following exposures:

The Plague[1]

The bombing of Hiroshima[2]

The atmospheric testing of nuclear weapons[3]

The Love Canal contamination[4]

The PBB contamination of Michigan cattle feed[5]

The PCB contamination of Japanese cooking oil[6]

The occupational exposure of industrial employees to toxic chemicals[7]

The Three Mile Island accident[8]

The criteria used for choosing these studies were: (1) they are social science studies of the invisible exposures as such, and (2) they take a broad perspective and look at several aspects of the exposure in question. In addition, several studies that looked only at particular aspects of a given invisible exposure were also used in putting together the synthesis found in this book.

There is one study that I have not drawn on at any length in preparing this book, even though it meets the two criteria mentioned above. It is Reich's study of the Seveso, Italy, accident involving dioxin.[9] I did not include the Seveso study because the exposure it describes was a very complicated situation that, while consistent with the findings of this book, raises issues that could not be dealt with adequately here. Some of the better-known Three Mile Island studies have also been excluded because they did not study any of the phenomena with which this book is concerned.[10]

In essence, then, *Invisible Trauma* is a preliminary comparative analysis of the several case studies that have been done to date of the psychological effects of the invisible contaminants. It is preliminary in that: (1) there have been, thus far, only a small number of studies on which one can draw in making this analysis, and (2) only a limited portion of the various psychosocial consequences of the invisible exposures have been examined at this point. Nevertheless, there is still much to be learned by pursuing the inquiry now.

An invisible exposure generates a fairly complex sequence of events. In the wake of an invisible exposure an equilibrated system, if you will, develops that involves a fairly constant cast of characters. The creation of this system is initiated by the occurrence of the exposure. In the wake of the exposure, there develops a political and scientific dialogue about what the health effects of that exposure have been and will be. Almost invariably, these conflicted dialogues remain unresolved; dwindling down to a steady and unconcluded state. In case after case, one finds that there is little or no scientific and/or political agreement as to what the effects of the exposure are or will be.

The participating parties to the usual postexposure dialogue are as follows:

The exposed population

The contaminating institutions

The involved regulatory institutions

The scientific community

The public health and private medical communities

Local governments

The federal government

The political groups that form in response to the exposure

The legal community

The press

Within the complicated dynamic that develops between these various groups, *Invisible Trauma* focuses on the psychological consequences of an invisible exposure for those people in the exposed population who come to believe that they have been, or might have been, physically injured by that exposure. It is this group of people that will attempt to adapt to the health threats posed by an invisible contamination. What these people discover, in the process of attempting to cope with the health effects of these exposures, is that they have inherited a most difficult task. The difficulty of their endeavor arises in consequence of the environmental and medical invisibility of the involved contaminants. (See chapter 3 for definition of environmental and medical invisibility.)

Ironically, it is the adaptational dilemmas that exposees encounter, in the process of attempting to adapt to an invisible exposure, that lead to the development of the psychological traumas of an invisible contamination. This book describes these traumata and analyzes the process by which a person's attempts to adapt to an invisible exposure can give rise to the problems that such exposures generate.

2
The Plague

E ven the most conservative figures make it abundantly clear how great and devastating an impact the medieval Plague had upon its helpless victim: Europe. In the middle of the fourteenth century, just prior to the onslaught of the Plague, Europe had a population of approximately 100 million.[1] The most conservative estimates tell us that 25 million people died of plague in the first four years that the disease raged in Europe.[2] One out of every four Europeans died of plague between 1347 and 1351.

Many believe that plague mortality was considerably higher. The well-known and respected papal physician Guy de Chauliac estimated that 75 million Europeans succumbed to the medieval Plague.[3] Given the dimensions of plague mortality, it is easy to understand that the Plague was an event large enough to catch the attention and imagination of European society. The destruction and death that it sowed was a catalyst for several significant and enduring changes in the structure and fabric of European society.

It is generally held that the medieval Plague originated in the Kirghiz Steppes, which is now part of the southeastern underbelly of the Soviet Union. The modern Kirghiz Republic shares boundaries with China and Afghanistan, and its steppes were and still are a fertile breeding ground for wild rodents.

The disease probably left these steppes with a band of Mongolian Tartars, who had entered into an alliance with the Venetians toward the end of capturing the Crimean port of Caffa from the Genovese. The Venetians and Genovese were in competition for the then-emerging oriental trade, and the Venetians desired control of Caffa so that they might dominate trade in the Black Sea. Toward this end they basically contracted with the Tartars to lay siege to and destroy Caffa.

The Tartars came to Caffa directly from the Kirghiz Steppes, where they had been recently involved in other wars. They encircled Caffa, cut off its supplies, and began a prolonged siege of the town. Just as the siege was beginning to take its toll, Tartar soldiers began to die en masse of an unknown disease. The Tartar army decided to end its siege and to withdraw from the environs.

Before withdrawing, the Tartar commander committed a singularly spiteful act of biological warfare. It is thought that this single act is what brought the Plague to Europe. The Tartars took the catapults with which they had been bombarding the walls of Caffa and bombarded the city one last time. But instead of using their normal munitions, they loaded the catapults with the bodies of dead Tartar soldiers. The dead soldiers had succumbed to the Plague.

In consequence, the unsuspecting inhabitants of Caffa contracted the Plague as well. All that remained to bring the Plague to Europe was for the infected Genovese to return to their equally unsuspecting native Italy.

Had the Genovese understood the etiology of the Plague, or even its mechanism of transmission, the disease might never have reached Europe. However, it was impossible for the Genovese to have guessed that they were bringing to Europe a catastrophic infectious disease that would endure there for more than four centuries. The Plague is caused by a bacterial infection, and bacteria were not discovered until the nineteenth century.

Specifically, the Plague is caused by the bacterium *Pasteurella pestis*. In nature, Plague is found as a disease of wild rodents such as rats, squirrels, and marmots. The Plague bacillus is transmitted from rodents to humans by a flea known as *Xenopsylla cheopis,* which makes its home in the hair of rodents.

It is believed that at Caffa the Plague was transmitted from the Tartars to the Genovese by the following sequence of events: first, the rats of Caffa ate the deceased and unattended Tartars. Then the fleas, in the process of feeding off of the now-contaminated rats, acquired the plague bacillus. The fleas, in turn, transmitted the plague bacillus to the Genovese by biting them.

The Plague has three different but overlapping clinical forms: (1) bubonic plague, (2) pneumonic plague, and (3) septicemic plague. All three forms are caused by the *Pasteurella pestis* bacterium, but they differ from one another in clinical presentation and area of involvement.

In bubonic plague, the primary site of infection is the lymph node. In fact, the name bubonic plague comes from the term bubo, a group of severely infected lymph nodes that are massively enlarged and filled with pus. These buboes are a constant feature of the bubonic form of plague, and they frequently open up to the skin and drain spontaneously. The symptoms of bubonic plague also include fever, prostration, and delirium. Death, when it occurs, usually happens during the first week of the illness.

Septicemic plague is an overwhelming infection of the blood stream. Usually it kills a person within days. Death almost always occurs before the infection has had time to localize in either the lymph nodes or the lungs. The symptoms of septicemic plague are virtually the same as those of bubonic plague except that there are no buboes in septicemic plague and the illness progresses more rapidly to death.

Pneumonic plague is a form of pneumonia, that is, it is an infection of the lung. It is characterized by the symptoms of pneumonia: a cough producing blood-tinged sputum, shortness of breath, cyanosis, and considerable prostration. Pneumonic plague can be spread from human to human, and it usually runs a fatal course within one to five days. All three forms of plague can now be successfully treated with antibiotics.

But in the fourteenth century Europe and its physicians were powerless in the face of the Plague. People were almost invariably killed by the infection. Death was quick, but it was not merciful. If you contacted bubonic plague, death typically came within five days of the first appearance of symptoms. The pneumonic form of the Plague took about three days to complete its task.

In the words of Guy de Chauliac, "It was useless and shameful for the doctors." For all intents and purposes, the Plague was, for the medieval physician, a disease caused by an invisible agent. It was an uncontrollable disaster that had been brought about by a wholly undiscernible state of affairs.

However, not everyone responded to the situation as though it were hopelessly beyond the realm of human control. In response to this most tangible of diseases, with its most invisible and intangible of causes, several theories on the etiology of the Plague were put forth by both the learned and unlearned men of the day. In turn, these theories spawned a large and imaginative gamut of measures designed to prevent the spread of the disease. Something had to be done. At least, people had to try to give the impression that something could be done.

Eventually, four major learned theories appeared regarding the causes of the Plague: (1) a not-unexpected theological theory that it was God's punishment for man's sins, (2) a theory regarding a "corruption of the air" that was believed to have its origins in a rather anthropocentric series of astronomical events, (3) an astrological theory that involved a multiple planetary conjunction, and (4) a theory based on the then-influential Galenic model of disease, that the Plague was a consequence of a humoral imbalance in the sick person's body.[4]

To the modern sensibility the medieval theories of the Plague are both amusing and incredible. Nonetheless, they represent the real attempts of responsible people to fight a terrible epidemic that was both beyond their control and caused by an agent invisible to their knowledge. By examining these theories from this vantage point, and by taking a careful look at the cognitive response of medieval Europeans to the Plague, one can perhaps learn something important about the modern mind.

In fourteenth-century Europe, France was thought to be the medical center of the world. The most prestigious medical institution of the day was the College of Physicians of the University of Paris. In 1348 King Philip of France requested of this royal college both an explanation of the causes of the Plague and a remedy for the devastating effects it was having. The college responded with a treatise known as the Paris Consultation. Anna Campbell summarizes that treatise as follows:

> The University of Paris, however, leader at the time in astronomical science, according to Duhem, and stronghold for Christendom of orthodox theology, boldly faced the problem, setting forth a confident explanation of how the conjunction of 1345 brought pestilence upon the Earth. On March 20, 1345, at one o'clock in the afternoon, occurred an important conjunction of three higher planets in the sign of Aquarius, which, with other conjunctions and eclipses, is the cause of the pernicious corruption of the surrounding air, as well as a sign of mortality, famine and other catastrophes not connected with the present subject. Aristotle is quoted and other, unnamed, ancient philosophers referred to for the fact that the conjunction of Saturn and Jupiter brings about the death of peoples and the depopulation of kingdoms, great accidents occurring on account of the change of the two stars themselves; and Albert of Cologne is adduced in support of the assertion that the conjunction of Mars and Jupiter causes great pestilence in the air, especially when it takes place in a warm and humid sign, as occurred in this instance. For, the Paris doctors explain, Jupiter, a warm and humid planet, drew up evil vapors from earth and water, and Mars, being excessively hot and dry, set fire to those vapors. Whence there were in the air flashes of lightning, lights, pestilential vapors, and fires, especially since Mars, a malevolent planet generating choler and wars, was from the sixth of October, 1347, to the end of May of the present year in the lion together with the head of the dragon. Not only did all of them, as they are warm, attract many vapors, but Mars, being on the wane, was very active in this respect, and also, turning toward Jupiter its evil aspect, engendered a disposition or quality hostile to human life. From this were generated strong winds, which, according to Albert, Jupiter has the property of raising, particularly, from the south, giving rise in lower countries to very great heat and dampness; in regions about Paris the dampness was greater than the heat.[5]

The central idea here is that astronomical events caused a fouling of the atmosphere that, in turn, caused the Plague. This explanation was adopted by authorities all over Europe. The idea that epidemics were caused by "corruption of the air" in fact predated the Parisian consultation. It was the conception of the etiology of epidemics that had come down to medieval European medicine from Hippocrates and Galen.

The Italian rendering of this theory, which can be found in the *Annales Pistorienses,* is more accessible than the French version and thus also worthy of consideration. I quote, once again, from Anna Campbell's summary of its contents:

In India and about the Great Sea, constellations, combating the rays of the sun, struggled violently with the waters of that sea, which rose in vapor and fell again for twenty-eight days. At last the greater part of them were drawn up as vapors, those which were left being so corrupted that the fish within them died. The corrupted vapors which had been drawn out could not be consumed by the sun, nor could they be converted into wholesome water like hail and dew, but spread abroad through the air. This had happened in Arabia, India, Crete, Macedonia, Hungary, Albania and Sicily, and if it should reach Sardinia no one would survive: the danger would continue in countries to which this air had access as long as the sun was in the sign of the lion. But the constellations were by their divine might striving to aid the human race, and, together with the sun, to break through the mists; so that within the next ten days the mists would be changed into noisome rain, purifying the air. From this rain people should protect themselves, and before and after it build large fires in open public places and in their places.[6]

The earthquake of 1347 was another oft-mentioned medieval theory of the cause of the Plague. The earthquake theory was also related to the air-corruption hypothesis. A treatise of unknown authorship, entitled *It Is from Divine Wrath That the Mortality of These Years Proceeds,* held that the earthquake of 1347 had corrupted the air, as earthquakes were then thought to do, and thus had caused the Plague.[7]

Medieval scholars believed that earthquakes were caused by "the exhalation of fumes caught up in the earth's inner parts." These fumes were thought to beat against the insides of the earth's surface, causing the earth to shake. Apparently, some of these geological fumes were thought to have escaped into the atmosphere during the earthquake of 1347, generally fouling and corrupting the air. This atmospheric corruption led, of course, to the Plague epidemic.

The previously mentioned Parisian Consultation also noted that the earthquake of 1347 had been a corrupter of the air and thus contributed to the Plague. The Italian physician Alfonso of Cordova held a similar view.

Corruption of the air, as a proximate cause of the Plague, was mentioned repeatedly in the learned treatises of the time. The well-regarded Moorish physician Ibn Khatimah, from the kingdom of Grenada, held that corruption of the air played a central role in causing the Plague. He believed that this disturbance of the air had been caused by: (1) the astronomical events mentioned in the Paris Consultation, (2) the recent irregularity of the seasons, and (3) the putrid fumes of decaying matter, including manure, stagnant water, swampy fields, rotting plants, and unburned corpses.[8]

Finally, the Italian physician Gentile of Foligno held that the Plague was caused by "perceptible corruptions" of either the air that was near at hand or the air that had been brought from the south by the wind. He believed that this defilement of the air occurred at the openings of wells and caverns that had been shut up for too long, as a result of the shutting up of air in roofs and walls, and on account of the stercus of animals, corpses, or other "evil smelling putrefactions." The good physician from Foligno also cautioned that people who had large pores were more susceptible to Plague than those with narrow pores. He held that this was because wider pores admitted more corrupted air into a person's body. In consequence of this analysis he recommended that people avoid taking hot baths. His rationale was, of course, that hot baths would open up the pores and render a person more vulnerable to contracting the Plague.[9] Given his premises, his recommendation is certainly logical.

The same judgment might also be passed on some of the other preventive remedies recommended by medieval experts. Flight from affected areas was recommended by all of the known medieval authorities who wrote on the Plague. The rationale was that a person leaving an epidemic area was avoiding exposure to the corrupt air that was pathologically present there.

If one were unable to flee, it was widely believed that one would do well to "rectify" the air in one's environment. Rectifying the air was thought to purify that atmosphere and eliminate the conditions that were causing the Plague.

The central concept in the process of rectifying corrupt air seems to have concerned changing its odor, an approach apparently derived from the belief that one of the cardinal properties of corrupted air was its foul odor. In consequence, it was believed that one could change a corrupted atmosphere into an incorrupt one by altering its odor. Standard procedure for accomplishing this was to introduce pleasant-smelling aromatic substances into the air.

Specifically, the idea developed that the air in one's dwellings could be purified by burning specific dry and odoriferous woods such as juniper, ash, rosemary, and pine. In winter, additional aromatic items such as amber, musk, cypress, laurel, and mastic were also to be burned. In summer, people were admonished to fill their houses with "cool, pleasant smelling" plants and flowers.

In a similar vein, means were prescribed by which people could protect themselves while walking around in the more treacherous public domains. The proper means for accomplishing this end was to carry around in one's hand either an apple or a piece of burning amber (depending upon one's financial means) and to smell it constantly as one walked about in public places.

It was also believed that one could improve the chances of survival by giving one's body the proper protective odor. People sprinkled themselves with citron and lemon juice and rubbed themselves with roses and violets.

Such were mainstream medieval notions as to how to protect oneself from contracting the Plague. To give one example of the circles in which these ideas were considered to have merit, it is known that the Pope Clement VI's physician burned large aromatic bonfires of the type described above and required the pope to sit among them while they burned.[10]

The pope seems to have had his own thoughts as to what was essential in these matters. He constantly wore an emerald ring that he believed would protect him from Plague-bearing vapors. Others believed that wearing a tiny image of a lion carved entirely of gold would protect a person from the Plague. In the pope's case, it seems likely that he survived because of his seclusion in his castle at Avignon.

Most people did not have the luxury of complete escape, and it will surprise no contemporary reader that none of the recommended preventive remedies, save flight, are known to have had any beneficial effect. The Plague raged on for four wanton years, thoroughly changing the social fabric of Europe. Giovanni Boccaccio wrote that all government, law enforcement, religious ceremony, and medical practice vanished. The people who had performed these tasks were either dead or afraid to carry them out.

The ranks of the priesthood were decimated. Many priests died as a consequence of giving last rites to dying victims of the Plague. Eventually, their death rates were so high that priests were no longer willing to administer the rites. For much the same reason, doctors also vanished and left the dying unattended.

Perhaps the most disconcerting social development was the oft-reported phenomenon that families literally deserted their sick members. In the words of Guy de Chauliac, "Father did not visit son, nor the son his father. Charity was dead and hope crushed."[11]

3
Invisibility and Ambiguity

Perhaps you are wondering about the relevance of the Plague in a book about the psychosocial effects of invisible environmental contaminants. The first of several answers is that for the inhabitants of medieval Europe, the Plague was caused by an invisible environmental contaminant: the *Pasteurella pestis* bacterium. Medieval scientists had absolutely no idea that any such thing as bacteria existed. Janssen had not yet invented the microscope. The concept of microbial infection had yet to be conceived or delineated. Pasteur had yet to establish the science of bacteriology, and no one knew anything at all about the diagnostic virtues of the gram stain. The ultimate consequence of these circumstances is that the Plague was a mystery to medieval Europeans. No one really knew what had brought this catastrophe to their doorsteps, and control of the Plague was far beyond the reach of the medieval European mind.

Modern industrial societies, for all of their scientific advancement and acuity, are also visited by invisible environmental contaminants. Most of today's invisible contaminants are the various forms of radiation and the toxic chemicals produced by the industrial processes that nurture our modern way of life. There are, to be certain, important differences between the health effects of the Plague and the health effects of industrial contamination. However, it is the similarity of their respective psychological effects that interests us. Before moving on to consider these similarities, let us establish a precise definition of the term invisible environmental contaminant.

An invisible environmental contaminant is a substance or energy form that is: (1) environmentally invisible and/or (2) medically invisible. To the extent that a contaminant is medically invisible, it will be invisible to physicians evaluating and treating patients exposed to the contaminant.

A contaminant is environmentally invisible if it is impossible for human beings to detect the presence of that contaminant with any of their senses. Ionizing radiation, for example, is environmentally invisible. It is not within the realm of the human sensory capacities to see, smell, taste, touch, or hear ionizing radiation. Thus it is quite impossible for humans to determine if and when they are being exposed to ionizing radiation.

The significance of environmental invisibility is that it makes it impossible for exposed or potentially exposed people to determine if they are in a dangerous situation. To be more precise, the environmental invisibility of a contaminant makes it impossible for exposed individuals to determine any of the following: (1) if they are in an environment in which the invisible contaminant is present, (2) whether a contaminant that is known to be present is actually being absorbed by the tissues of their bodies, (3) how large a dose of the contaminant they are absorbing, and (4) whether the absorbed dose is dangerous.

It can also be impossible to evaluate the danger of an invisible contaminant even when scientific instruments are used to detect its presence. For example, in the early stages of the Love Canal accident, the New York State Department of Health took air readings inside several of the homes bordering on the Love Canal toxic waste dump site. The purpose of these measurements was to assess the amount of toxic chemicals that had vaporized into the basements of the homes in question. Health department officials called a community meeting to announce the results of their tests. Residents were "handed mimeographed lists with the names of ten polysyllabic chemicals on them. Next to the chemical compounds were numbers representing values for air readings in their basements. The people's addresses were written in at the top of the sheets."[1]

After a brief silence, "the officials were immediately bombarded by questions from the residents. 'What do these numbers mean? We have a playroom—a family room—a bedroom—in the basement. Should we stop using it? Is the rest of my house safe?' The officials, who had probably not anticipated the questions, simply responded [over and over again] that they did not know the meanings of the raw figures. Their response increased the mistrust the residents were beginning to feel for their government officials."[2]

The situation is entirely different with visible contaminants. Imagine that you are standing on the street watching your house burn down. You would like to try and enter your house by the kitchen door to rescue your dog, who is stuck in the basement. As soon as you enter the kitchen, however, you realize that you've made a serious mistake. The smoke is so thick that it threatens to overcome you. You can feel the smoke in your lungs. As your head grows light, you begin to worry about losing your consciousness. Reluctantly admitting defeat, you turn and run out of your house.

In contrast to a situation involving an invisible contaminant, you could see, smell, and feel the smoke in your lungs. Because the smoke was both environmentally and medically visible, you immediately knew that you were in a dangerous situation and you adapted to it by taking measures to protect yourself. The invisibility of the invisible environmental contaminants makes adaptation to the threats they pose a much more difficult and imprecise matter.

An environmental contaminant is medically invisible if it causes disease and disease processes that are at some point invisible to either the lay or professional medical eye. For example, a liver cancer caused by an exposure to vinyl chloride will not become symptomatic, and thus clinically apparent, until several years after the exposure occurs. During the time between the original vinyl chloride exposure and the eventual clinical detection of the cancer that it has caused, the gestating cancer is not apparent to either the person in whom that cancer is growing or to the physicians who are caring for that person.

This period of time between the exposure to a contaminant and the clinical detection of the resultant disease is known as the latency period. The existence of this latency period is responsible for a form of medical invisibility called latency invisibility.

Ionizing radiation is another contaminant known to have a latency period. The diseases caused by radiation have latency invisibility because of the following circumstances: In the dose range in which radiation can cause delayed radiation illness (for example, cancer) the actual biological damage done at the time of exposure occurs at the cellular level. This early cellular damage is present in the form of either genetic mutations—which can lead to cancers or birth defects—or as one of several types of cytoplasmic injuries. These early cellular injuries can develop, over three to thirty-five years, into both the cancers and the many forms of nontumorous lesions caused by radiation.

During the latency period, it is generally impossible to detect the presence of early cellular lesions. Thus it is impossible for medical scientists to tell individuals who have been exposed to radiation whether or not they will develop a disease as a result of that exposure. This, then, is the biology of latency invisibility.

The second basic form of medical invisibility is etiological invisibility. An invisible environmental contaminant has etiological invisibility if it produces diseases or disease symptoms that cannot be attributed to the contaminant that has produced them. For example, leukemia is a disease that has been amply proven to result from ionizing radiation. The original and classic evidence for this causal connection comes from two groups of studies: (1) the Atomic Bomb Casualty Commission studies of the Hiroshima and Nagasaki survivors and (2) the British studies of the ankylosing spondylitis patients who were treated in the 1930s and 1940s with high doses of therapeutic x-rays to the cervical spine.

In spite of this ample epidemiological (that is, statistical) evidence that radiation causes leukemia, it remains impossible to prove that any given and specific case of leukemia has or has not been caused by an exposure to radiation. This etiological invisibility is a consequence of two facts: (1) there is no clinical pathology of radiation lesions and (2) there are other causes of leukemia.

Clinical pathology is the field within medicine that is responsible for the laboratory evaluation and diagnosis of diseases. For example, clinical pathology gives medicine the tools and techniques to determine the type of microorganism (bacteria, virus, fungus, and so on) that is causing a given case of infectious disease. In the case of a meningitis, this is done by examining a patient's cerebrospinal fluid, which is obtained by doing a lumbar puncture (spinal tap). By examining and culturing the spinal fluid, pathologists can determine the exact microorganism that is causing the meningitis in question. Physicians need this type of information to treat the meningitis patient with the correct antimicrobial drug.

There is no clinical pathology of radiation lesions because at the present there are no laboratory techniques that can be used to analyze diseases caused by radiation. For example, it would be impossible to scientifically demonstrate that a leukemia found in a survivor of the bombing of Hiroshima was definitely caused by the radiation released by that bomb. The problem comes down to this fact: there is no morphological or biochemical *marker* that distinguishes the diseased white blood cells of a leukemia caused by radiation from the diseased white blood cells of a leukemia caused by some other agent. There is no method for distinguishing whether a given case of leukemia has been caused by radiation or by benzene or by some other agent.

Two factors in addition to the absence of a contaminant-specific clinical pathology can result in etiological invisibility. They are: (1) a lack of awareness that the responsible invisible contaminant exists and (2) a lack of awareness of a causal relationship between a given contaminant and the disease(s) that it produces.

The historical situation at the time of the medieval Plague is an example of the first type of predicament. Any number of causal relationships between contaminant and disease—vinyl chloride and hepatic angiosarcoma, cigarette smoking and lung cancer, diethylstilbestrol and vaginal cancer, and asbestos and mesothelioma—are examples of the second predicament. In each of these examples, there was a long period during which the causal relationship between the contaminant and the disease it produced went unrecognized.

A dilemma that is akin to but different from medical invisibility is the phenomenon of diagnostic ambiguity. A formal definition of diagnostic ambiguity is the presentation in a patient of somatic symptoms that the patient and that patient's physicians are unable to diagnose. An excellent example of temporary diagnostic ambiguity involving an invisible environmental contaminant can be found in the polychlorinated biphenyl (PCB) contamination of cooking oil in western Japan, which has been described by M.R. Reich.[3]

The contamination persisted for nine months before it was detected. It first occurred in February of 1968, and retrospective analysis indicates that people began to get ill from the contamination at least as early as March 1968. However, the contamination produced a cluster of symptoms that was not known at the time to be caused by PCB intoxication or even to exist as a diagnostic entity. The symptoms of this PCB poisoning were loss of appetite, fatigue, puffy eyelids, headaches, limb pain, excessive eye secretions, decreased visual acuity, and severe chloracne.

"Throughout the summer of 1968, the Kamino family [a family suffering from PCB contamination] sought help from one doctor after another. 'No one knew what the cause was . . . all the doctors said "It's a strange disease." We knew that the disease was something different, something strange, never before seen or experienced. . . . but we did not have any idea who was responsible for our disease.' Kamino sensed that if the doctors could not name the disease, then the patient must somehow be at fault."[4]

By October 1968 Japanese physicians had begun to understand that the commercial contamination of rice oil with PCB was causing a public health problem among the population of western Japan. Recognition came when the syndrome of PCB symptoms was identified as a diagnostic entity and given the name Yusho. From then on the diagnostic ambiguity of this PCB-caused illness ceased to exist.

The diagnostic ambiguity in the Yusho episode was a consequence of the fact that when the contamination began, medical science was unaware that PCB exposure could cause a disease entity with the symptoms of Yusho. Consequently, individual physicians were not familiar with the fact that PCB could cause Yusho. This diagnostic category was simply not available to or a part of their diagnostic inquiries. Consequently, the diagnosis could not be made.

One sees similar situations of diagnostic ambiguity in many illnesses involving an invisible contamination. The similarity between medical invisibility and diagnostic ambiguity creates the temptation to call this one phenomenon — diagnostic invisibility — instead of two. But this would be incorrect.

The temptation arises from the fact that diagnostic ambiguity as a result of incomplete scientific knowledge seems to derive, at least in part, from both the latency and etiological invisibilities of the various diseases produced by an invisible contaminant. After all, an unseen disease that becomes clinically apparent months or years after an invisible exposure is quite difficult to relate empirically to the contaminant that has caused it. In addition, there is a sense in which a disease is invisible if it has not been diagnosed.

To have called this phenomenon diagnostic invisibility would have destroyed the meaning of the word invisible. Both latency and etiological invisibility involve a literal invisibility — the nonappearance of some aspect of the disease process in question. Latency invisibility involves the nonappearance of symptoms, and etiological invisibility involves the nonappearance of an etiological marker. Diagnostic ambiguity does not involve a nonappearance. It involves the absence of a diagnostic, or conceptual, category in the presence of apparent somatic symptoms.

In addition to this problem with the meaning of the word, diagnostic ambiguity can also be caused by a number of other circumstances, which may or may not be related to an exposure to an invisible contaminant. Such situations include (1) atypical presentations of known diagnostic entities, (2) the presentation of idiosyncratic psychosomatic symptoms, and (3) the presentation of hypochondriacal symptoms. In each of these situations a physician may be unable to find a diagnostic category for a patient's somatic or somatoform symptoms. Given that the essence of diagnostic ambiguity is the absence of a diagnostic category, and that there are a number of situations unrelated to invisible contaminants in which a diagnostic category cannot be adduced, it would be inaccurate to call this phenomenon a form of medical invisibility.

But one common thread does connect environmental invisibility, medical invisibility, and diagnostic ambiguity. The thread is that all three conditions render it difficult, if not impossible, for a person to adapt empirically to the dangers posed by an exposure to an invisible contaminant. Herein lies the significance of the invisibility and ambiguity that adhere to the invisible environmental contaminants. The invisibility and ambiguity of the invisible contaminants present the exposed person with two basic adaptive dilemmas.

The first dilemma is that it is virtually impossible to assess and protect oneself from the dangers of exposure to an invisible contaminant. It is most difficult to protect oneself from a threat that one cannot see. There is no way for a person to ascertain, in the presence of an invisible threat, whether or not he or she is in a dangerous situation. There is no warning of danger, no indication that a dangerous exposure is occurring, and no immediate indication that bodily damage is being done. There is no smoke to be seen, and nothing like the symptoms of smoke inhalation.

A second dilemma is that the ambiguity and invisibility of the diseases caused by invisible contaminants makes it difficult to obtain medical care for illnesses caused by an invisible exposure. A person who has contracted an invisible disease does not even know that he or she needs medical care. Patients who present to a physician with undiagnosable somatic symptoms will be deprived of an understanding of and treatment for their illness.

In summary, the person exposed to an invisible environmental contaminant faces two basic adaptive dilemmas: (1) how to protect himself or herself from the actual *exposure* to the contaminant and (2) how to protect himself or herself from the *health effects* of that exposure. These adaptive dilemmas can in turn generate an awesome amount of uncertainty for the exposed individual. Not only is this uncertainty a problem in and of itself, but it can also become the nidus of unwanted and enduring cognitive, emotional, and behavioral change.

4

The Speculative Response to Invisible Contamination

The second basic relevancy of the Plague to our investigation of the psychosocial effects of the invisible environmental contaminants is to be found in the speculative response of both the learned and unlearned Europeans to the disease. Despite the Plague's etiological invisibility, and despite the fact that nobody really knew what was causing the epidemic, there was no lack of authoritative pronouncements about its origins. The highly esteemed Paris College of Physicians appears to have put forth its astronomical theory of atmospheric pollution as if there was no doubt of its veracity.

Four major theories eventually appeared regarding the causes of the Plague.[1] These are the Parisian theory that the disease was caused by foul atmosphere, the theological theory that the disease was a punishment from God,[2] the astrological theory that the disease was caused by celestial bodies, and the medical theory that the disease was caused by an imbalance of bodily humors.

The appearance of these four particular theories at the time of the Plague constitutes confirmation of Lazarus's hypothesis that "the more ambiguous are the stimulus clues concerning the nature of anticipated [threat], the more important are general belief systems in determining the appraisal process [of that threat]."[3] One sees, in the learned medieval appraisal of the causes of the Plague, the projection, if you will, of several of the more important systematic belief systems of that time: (1) the classical model of epidemics in the Parisian theory, (2) Catholic theology in the theological model, (3) astrology, as found in the astrological model, and (4) the classical model of medicine, once again, as found in the humoral theory of the Plague.

Imagine a whole continent beset by the Plague. Imagine being confronted by an uncontrollable epidemic that was killing at least one in every four persons. It was clearly a matter that could not be easily or advantageously ignored. Unfortunately, in a cultural milieu in which empirical knowledge of the etiology of the Plague was impossible, there was not much that could be done. The development of a public health program that could successfully prevent and treat the Plague epidemic was, from the very beginning, an impossibility.

What one sees, then, in these medieval theories regarding the causes of the Plague is an attempt to adapt to a threatening situation in which successful adaptation was simply not possible. Successful adaptation to the Plague was precluded because the causes of the Plague were not yet visible to the European eye. Nonetheless, medieval and renaissance physicians did not shy away from the task of attempting to explain and prevent the Plague. As we have already seen, theories were developed, and measures were taken.

The situation faced by medieval Europe is not unique to prescientific societies. The appearance of invisible and thus uncontrollable illness is not an infrequent occurrence in the industrial age. Confrontation with invisible and thus uncontrollable health problems can be found at the heart of many contemporary exposures to the invisible environmental contaminants.

Consider, for example, Fowlkes and Miller's description of the circumstances that occurred during the Love Canal disaster:

> In contrast, then, to natural disasters, which leave no doubt that a destructive event has occurred, the nature of what, exactly, occurred at Love Canal was, and continues to be, highly ambiguous. First, no visible event or impact occurred to which the larger society or the community qua community could bear witness. Second, the assertion by the New York State Department of Health that an emergency existed in the area did not (and, indeed, could not) derive from the comprehensive documentation of the exact impact of chemical exposure on the population. The circumstances at Love Canal were such that no real evidence, either self-ascertained or expert-based, confirmed the occurrence of a disaster. Neither was there evidence to disconfirm the occurrence of a disaster. Indeed, the possibility that life threatening conditions prevailed in the neighborhood had been strongly suggested by officials and clearly recognized by the citizens.[4]

In other words, the residents of Love Canal did not have reliable information with which they could determine whether or not they were in a dangerous situation. They did not really know whether they needed to protect themselves from the chemicals buried at Love Canal. And like medieval Europeans contending with the Plague, they were also unable to obtain information with which to protect themselves should that be necessary.

As described by Fowlkes and Miller, this information was simply not available. This was true in spite of the fact that we live in an era that is veritably teeming with the scientific and technological tools that one would think should make such information available.

This type of adaptive dilemma is by no means unique in modern times to the Love Canal accident. It has actually been a characteristic occurrence in all of the studied exposures involving invisible environmental contaminants.

Dilemmas of this type, in which the information necessary for successful adaptation to an invisible exposure is not available, have been experienced and documented in the aftermath of (1) the Three Mile Island accident,[5] (2) military participation in atmospheric nuclear weapons tests,[6] (3) an industrial accident that resulted in significant dioxin contamination of the Italian community of Seveso,[7] (4) a PBB contamination of livestock feed in Michigan,[8] (5) a PCB contamination of cooking oil in western Japan,[9] and (6) a methyl alcohol contamination of illegally distilled whiskey in Atlanta.[10]

The point that I would like to make is this: the cognitive response to all of these modern contaminants is much the same as the medieval response to the Plague. In each of these situations involving an exposure to invisible contaminants—whether in scientific or prescientific societies—one finds that invisible health threats are met by the development of nonempirical belief systems about the nature of the threats.

A belief system is a coherent collection of beliefs that together portray a description of reality. All of our notions of reality are embodied and manifest in our belief systems about the nature of the universe and ourselves. The theory of evolution and the creationist view of our origins are both belief systems.

Empirical belief systems are those deduced from the observation of natural events in accordance with the strictures of the scientific method. Nonempirical belief systems are deductions based on data that are qualitatively or quantitatively inadequate from a scientific perspective.

In the instance of an invisible contaminant, there is a paucity of information about the effects of exposure because of its invisibility. Such conditions are breeding grounds for the creation of nonempirical belief systems. For example, when the Department of Defense contends that an atomic veteran's cancer is unrelated to a previous radiation exposure, it is making a nonempirical assessment to the etiology of that cancer. It is absolutely impossible to empirically prove or disprove the implied hypothesis. No known marker indicates whether or not a given case of leukemia has been caused by a radiation exposure.

The boundary between empirical and nonempirical belief systems is sometimes imprecise. For example, the history of science is littered with theories that were accepted as good science in their time only to be discarded, at a later date, as being scientifically incorrect. Baron George Cuvier's Catastrophe Theory is an easy example. Cuvier's theory, which was well received in his own time, attempted to reconcile eighteenth century fossil findings with the Biblical version of creation.

In a similar manner, it would be incorrect to say that the reality depicted by a nonempirical belief system is necessarily true or false. Once again, to say that a belief system is nonempirical is only to say that it is based on insufficient data. Nonempirical belief systems can appear to be either correct or incorrect. The Plague theories at which we have been looking appear, with the benefit of six centuries of hindsight, to be preposterous.

On the other hand, the conclusions reached by farmers living in the Three Mile Island area appear to have some basis in observed fact. Immediately after the accident, many of these farmers experienced an increased incidence of illness and reproductive problems in their livestock. Many of them concluded, on the basis of this observed temporal contiguity, that their livestock problems had been caused by the radiation released during the accident. The sequence of events is, indeed, suggestive, and the farmers may have even been correct. But at the time, sufficient data was not available to warrant the conclusions they had reached.

To reiterate, to say that a belief system is a nonempirical belief system is not to say that the beliefs it contains are incorrect or dishonest. As we shall be seeing, in the instance of an invisible exposure, nonempirical belief systems are constructed as a means of having a cognitive ground from which one can adapt to the threats posed by that exposure.

The construction of nonempirical belief systems in consequence of a modern exposure to an invisible contaminant has been well documented. Fowlkes and Miller[11] found that Love Canal residents constructed beliefs about the dangers posed by the toxic chemicals released from the Love Canal. Levine[12] found that Love Canal residents had constructed a belief system about the nature of the problem and about how it could be best resolved. I have described belief systems developed by both military veterans of our atmospheric nuclear weapons testing programs[13] and by residents of the Three Mile Island area.[14] Belief systems in both of these populations centered around the health effects of their exposures to radiation. Finally, Brodsky has documented the construction of belief systems in workers occupationally exposed to toxic chemicals.

This phenomenon, the creation of nonempirical belief systems in response to invisible health threats, is not unique to the societies of Western civilization. The anthropological literature provides abundant examples of this type of cognitive response to invisible medical threats, suggesting that it might somehow comprise a basic form of human cognitive response to the uncontrollable illnesses caused by invisible pathological processes.

One example from the anthropological literature comes from Francis L.K. Hsu's observations of a cholera epidemic in the small town of Hsi Ch'eng in southwestern China.[15]

At the time of the epidemic, Hsi Ch'eng was a rural market town of 8,000 people. The town's elevation is 6,700 feet. The principal occupation of the area was agriculture, and the staple crop was rice.

In the spring of 1942, a serious cholera epidemic engulfed Hsi Ch'eng. Between May 10 and June 10 two hundred people died of cholera in the town. Funeral processions became a common sight, and the epidemic weighed heavily on the spirit of the survivors. Hsu describes a town in which the "men and women became reticent and gloomy." Night life disappeared.

Cholera, like the Plague, is caused by bacteria. The particular bacterium that causes cholera is known as *Vibrio comma.* Cholera is spread primarily by the fecal contamination of food and water. The symptoms of cholera are severe diarrhea, severe dehydration, and death.

Cholera has been historically known and feared in all parts of China. The traditional Chinese explanation for cholera—a disease caused by what was for them an invisible etiological agent—is that it is caused by epidemic-carrying spirits. It is believed that these spirits are sent at the behest of the gods when the people have affronted them with immoral behavior.

In 1942, despite the presence of a modern Western hospital and physician in Hsi Ch'eng, the vast majority of the town's inhabitants took no interest in either the educational programs or free medical care offered by the hospital for prevention and treatment of cholera. For townspeople, the causes of cholera were to be found in the supernatural realm. Viewed from this perspective, going to a Western hospital was of limited value.

The town regarded prayer meetings as the most important measure that could be taken to propitiate the gods. Nineteen prayer meetings were held during the month of the epidemic. The meetings were essentially occasions during which "priests prayed to the gods to forgive misconduct and exhorted the populace to be moral." These meetings were held round the clock, and one of them lasted six and a half days.

Posters were displayed throughout Hsi Ch'eng encouraging everyone to abstain from sex and to purge themselves of evil thought. A general effort was made to clear the town so that it would be pleasing to the gods' eyes. Taboos were placed on the consumption of foods including string beans, potatoes, pea curd, meat, fish, all sour fruits, and all confections.

The South African anthropologist Cassell has described a similar response amongst the Zulu to Western medical treatment for tuberculosis.[16] Tuberculosis is also caused by a bacterium.

> According to the Zulus, any disease associated with labored breathing, pains in the chest, loss of weight and [the] coughing up [of] bloodstained sputum [which are the commonest symptoms of pulmonary tuberculosis] as attributed to the machinations of an illwisher. This person causes poison to be put in the victim's food; he may do this personally or through the services of a familiar over whom he has control. The poison is not excreted through the bowel but remains indefinitely in the stomach causing a person to vomit blood and lose weight. Eventually, the influence of the poison affects the lungs and causes pains in the chest. The treatment consists in taking an emetic specifically prepared by a "witch-doctor" skilled in treating the disease. Once the emetic causes the poison to be vomited, the patient will be cured.

The Zulus apparently believe that tuberculosis was present in their society before their interactions with white colonials. However, Cassell writes,

> objective evidence . . . indicates that tuberculosis was extremely rare, if not absent, among the Zulus and other Bantu tribes until comparatively recent times. In discussing the history of tuberculosis in South Africa, one authority has this to say: "Up to the time of Livingstone who in his *Travels and Researchers in South Africa* states categorically that tuberculosis did not exist among the tribes, there is no evidence that clinically recognizable tuberculosis among the Bantu was other than a rarity." It is likely that this syndrome originally was produced by cases of pneumonia and congestive heart failure.[17]

It appears that Zulu beliefs about tuberculosis were either constructed at the time that tuberculosis was introduced into their tribe, or existed as an older belief that was generalized to apply to tuberculosis when it became prevalent. In either case, the belief was constructed in response to an uncontrollable illness caused by a pathogen invisible to the Zulu mind.

Another example of a nonempirical belief system that developed in response to an invisible health threat is the nineteenth-century belief—widely held in Europe and America—that tuberculosis descended upon individuals because they had a particular type of temperament. Susan Sontag took jaundiced note of this phenomenon in *Illness and Metaphor*—her diatribe against the similar ascription of a psychological etiology to the cancers. The tuberculosis bacillus, which is extremely difficult to culture, was invisible until it was discovered by Robert Koch in 1882. Until then it was generally held that tuberculosis was a disease of the melancholy, indolent, and repressed soul.

It appears that the development of nonempirical belief systems as a cognitive response to invisible and thus uncontrollable health threats may well be a phenomenon that occurs in all cultures and at all times. Perhaps what is at play here is a general principle of human behavior. Because this principle is an important point of departure for this discussion of the psychosocial effects of the invisible environmental contaminants, I would like to give it a name and state it in concise and hypothetical form. I would like to tentatively name it the medical uncertainty hypothesis and state it thus: when confronted with an invisible threat to one's health, some people will construct nonempirical belief systems as a form of knowledge about that threat.

It is tempting to dismiss this type of cognitive adaptation to invisible medical threats as nonsense. After all, this is not a form of scientifically informed adaptation. But sometimes the scientific information necessary for an adaptation to an invisible threat is simply not available.

This was certainly the case at Three Mile Island when, at the time of the accident, residents were faced with the decision of whether or not to evacuate the area. In the face of an invisible radiological threat to their health, TMI area residents sought out governmental and scientific authorities to determine if they were in a dangerous situation. They found that the various authorities gave answers that contradicted one another and at times themselves. Realizing that they could trust neither their own senses nor the appropriate authorities, many people made nonempirical decisions about the radiological dangers of Three Mile Island.

In this book we are interested in whether the nonempirical belief systems developed in response to an invisible health threat are adaptive or maladaptive. Can they have any adaptive value, and under what conditions can such systems become maladaptive? Before attempting to answer these questions, we will take a further, in-depth look at the situations that develop in consequence of an invisible exposure.

5
Introduction to Case Studies

T he complexity of the situations that can develop as a consequence of an invisible exposure is really beyond anticipation. The complexity is a function of the many uncertainties that can and do develop once exposure to an invisible contaminant has occurred. In the wake of an invisible exposure, a number of characteristic and important issues invariably arise and obstinately defy empirical resolution.

Sometimes resolution is impossible because the requisite studies have not been done or will take too long to do. On other occasions, science is simply unable to uncover the relevant information. In the same sense that there was no way for medieval Europeans to know what was really causing the Plague, it is often impossible for our society to answer important health-impact questions that develop after an exposure involving an invisible contaminant.

Conceptual presentation alone cannot do justice to the wealth of difficult and unanswerable questions that arise for all of the participants involved in an invisible exposure. Accordingly, it seems best to begin this presentation of the psychosocial effects of the invisible environmental contaminants with the presentation of three case studies. These case studies should serve to introduce the consistent patterns present in the chaotic and multifaceted milieu that an invisible exposure creates.

First I would like to present a simple descriptive model of the early phases of response by a person concerned about an invisible exposure. Basically, two different types of event can cause a person to become concerned about the personal effects of an invisible exposure. The first is simply the awareness that one is being exposed or has been exposed to an invisible pathogen. At Three Mile Island, for example, many people became deeply concerned about the health effects of the accident well before it was possible for TMI-caused radiogenic illness to become manifest. The fact of the exposure itself caused concern. The same thing happened at Love Canal, to name just one instance involving a chemical exposure.

It is important to note that not all invisible exposures generate this kind of compelling concern. For example, most people give little or no thought to the health effects of a diagnostic chest x-ray and few people are actively concerned about the health effects of the omnipresent industrial and automotive air pollution found in our large urban centers.

In addition, different people react differently to the same invisible exposure. Roughly 60 percent of the people living within five miles of Three Mile Island thought the situation was dangerous and evacuated the area during the accident; 40 percent thought the situation was safe enough to remain behind.[1] A survey taken three years after the accident found that 75.2 percent of the population living within five miles believed that "people living in the TMI area at the time of the accident were exposed to radiation." The remaining 24.8 percent thought that TMI residents had not received dangerous doses at the time of the accident.[2]

We have not yet studied in any systematic fashion what situational and personality variables cause individuals to become actively concerned about the health effects of an endured invisible exposure. Further research in this area would be important and welcomed. However, both social scientists and members of the general public are already well aware that situations do occur in which large numbers of people become concerned about the potential health effects of an invisible exposure. Fourteen thousand people who wanted to know if they were suffering from PCB contamination reported to public health clinics in western Japan after the Japanese government announced that a PCB contamination of cooking oil had occurred.[3] Four hundred and thirty-three people reported to one hospital's emergency room in Atlanta seeking to ascertain whether they were the victims of a methyl alcohol contamination of illegally distilled whiskey.[4] Finally, 50 to 60 percent of the approximately forty thousand people living within five miles of Three Mile Island left the area during the nuclear power plant accident there.[5] They thought that the radiation that had been or was about to be released from the plant was dangerous.

So the first type of event that will generate concern about an invisible contaminant is an actual exposure to one of those contaminants. A second precipitant of concern about invisible environmental contaminants is the occurrence of significant illness in a person who has had a history of an invisible exposure. Such a conjunction can cause a person to become deeply concerned about the health effects of a previous exposure. The association of significant illness and an invisible exposure can lead a previously exposed person to wonder whether the two events are related. It can also open the door for the exposed person to think about whether he or she will be developing future illnesses as a result of that previous exposure; and such questions seem to invariably lead to further concerns about detecting and treating these diseases. This is particularly likely if the exposed person suspects that he or she may have a contaminant-caused illness that is in a latency period. Once again, it is worth emphasizing that these matters can and do become issues of grave concern for the exposed person.

This sequence of events has been seen among military participants in atmospheric nuclear tests, workers occupationally exposed to toxic chemicals, and farmers whose livestock were the primary victims of a PBB exposure. Again, it is not yet known in any systematic fashion why some people who find themselves in this situation become concerned, while others do not. In addition, it is not yet known what proportion of people in this situation will go on to become vigilant about the effects of a previous invisible exposure.

However, study of the atomic veterans has suggested that certain kinds of illness patterns may be associated with concern by exposed people. Three distinct illness patterns have been found to be associated with atomic veteran vigilance about past exposures to radiation: (1) cancer, (2) multiple occurrences of major systemic illnesses, and (3) undiagnosable somatic or somatoform symptoms.[6]

Once a person decides to attempt to adapt to the threats posed by an invisible contaminant, certain difficulties begin to arise. It proves immensely difficult to successfully cope with an invisible exposure. The information that a person needs to make sensible adaptive responses is frequently not available. Thus, it often happens that, as a consequence of trying to adapt to an invisible exposure, exposed persons can find themselves in a swamp of what we are calling adaptational dilemmas and experienced uncertainties.

A preliminary model of concerned exposee response to an invisible exposure in shown in figure 5–1. This diagram is a schematic presentation of the early consequences of attempted adaptation to an invisible exposure. As has already been discussed, concerns about an invisible exposure can be precipitated by either the exposure itself or the development of significant illness subsequent to the exposure. Once a person becomes concerned about an invisible exposure, he or she will attempt to become informed about the exposure and to protect himself or herself from it, which will mean different things in different situations. For example, a person who is being exposed to an invisible contaminant will usually attempt to terminate the exposure and

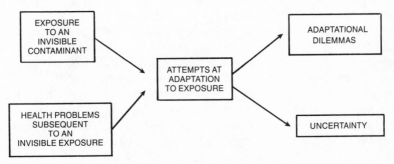

Figure 5–1. Adaptational Sequence #1

to evaluate its health effects. On the other hand, a person who has a history of radiation exposure and who subsequently is diagnosed as having precancerous lesion might well attempt to learn everything possible about the health effects of radiation and take extraordinary measures to monitor his or her health.

However, as the diagram suggests and as the case studies will amply demonstrate, these attempts at adaptation most often fail. These early adaptational failures often occur because of an insufficiency of information which can in turn be attributed to the environmental and medical invisibility of the involved contaminants.

As a result, attempts at coping with the threat of an invisible contamination almost inevitably lead the exposed person into a tangled and seemingly endless maze of uncertainties and adaptational dilemmas regarding the consequences of that exposure. The group of case studies that follows will illustrate this dynamic.

An experienced uncertainty is in this context an uncertainty as to the meaning of some aspect of an invisible exposure. For example, during the early days of the Three Mile Island accident, area residents were entirely uncertain about the significance of the radiological dangers posed by the accident. The accident itself was invisible and the radioactive materials that it released were also invisible. To further complicate matters, the various authorities and the media were giving contradictory reports about the radiological dangers. People did not know if they were being exposed to radiation, if they were being exposed to dangerous doses of radiation, or if, most important, they should evacuate the area to avoid new or additional exposures.

The phenomenon of the adaptational dilemma is very closely related to the experience of uncertainty. In the context of an invisible exposure, an adaptational dilemma is a situation in which a person finds that an empirically informed and thus satisfactory adaptation to an invisible exposure is not possible. That is, an adaptational dilemma is a situation in which a person is unable to determine how to adapt successfully to a threatening event or events. In the preceding example, the adaptational dilemma of the TMI residents was whether they should protect themselves from the radiation released from Three Mile Island by evacuating the area.

Adaptational dilemmas can also develop in response to the health effects of an exposure. If a person has been exposed to a contaminant with a latency period of several years, there is generally nothing that person can do to protect himself or herself from a potentially incubating disease until the contaminant-produced disease becomes symptomatic and thus clinically apparent. No protective adaptation can be made until it is too late.

Three case studies are presented in chapters 6 to 8. The first, a report of a PBB contamination of livestock feed in Michigan, is based on the work of Michael R. Reich.[7] The second, a study of the Love Canal disaster, leans heavily on the works of Adeline Levine, and Patricia Miller and Martha Fowlkes.[8] The final case is taken from my own research and is an in-depth portrait of the response of one military veteran to his exposure to radiation as a participant in two atmospheric nuclear weapons tests.[9]

These three case studies differ in two significant respects. The first is that the Love Canal and Michigan contaminations studies focus on the external events of an invisible exposure, while the third case study is a psychological portrait of one atomic veteran's response to the health problems he developed subsequent to his exposure to ionizing radiation.

The second difference is that the atomic veteran and Michigan case studies commence with the discovery of unexplained illness subsequent to an invisible exposure, and the Love Canal case study begins with the awareness that an invisible exposure is occurring. The significance of this later variation is that the particular dilemmas and uncertainties experienced by an exposed person differ to some extent according to the type of event that has precipitated concern about an invisible exposure.

A list of the various types of experienced uncertainties that can and do develop subsequent to an invisible exposure is presented below. Look for them as you read the case studies. Definition and extended discussion of each type of uncertainty are found in chapter 9. The typology of experienced uncertainties is as follows:

 1. previous exposure uncertainty
 2. present exposure uncertainty
 3. evacuation uncertainty
 4. boundary uncertainty
 5. dose uncertainty
 6. significance of dose uncertainty
 7. latency uncertainty
 8. etiological uncertainty
 9. diagnostic uncertainty
10. prognostic uncertainty
11. treatment uncertainty
12. coping uncertainty
13. financial uncertainty.

6
Michigan PBB Case Study

Michigan Chemical Corporation was a firm that produced a number of chemicals for commercial purposes. It began producing polybrominated biphenyls (PBB) in 1970 for use as a fire retardant in molded plastic parts. Typically, PBBs were used in the production of televisions, typewriters, and business machines. Michigan Chemical's brand name for this product was Firemaster BP-6.

In the early 1970s Dow and the DuPont corporations separately evaluated the toxicity of the PBB compounds and decided not to manufacture a PBB product. Both corporations publicly announced their decisions in 1972. The DuPont study found that PBBs cross the rat placenta, accumulate in fetal tissue, and cause significant liver damage. Dow's research program demonstrated that the PBBs can both accumulate in tissues and cause liver damage. Both corporations decided that the PBBs were too toxic to use for commercial purposes.

Nonetheless, Michigan Chemical continued to produce Firemaster BP-6. At the same time, it also produced a magnesium oxide product used as a sweet-for dairy cattle feed. Magnesium oxide is used as a feed additive because it results in increased feed consumption, which in turn produces increased milk and butterfat. Michigan Chemical's name for this additive was Nutrimaster.

Michigan Chemical normally used color-coded bags to package its products. The purpose of the color coding was to assure that the various products would not get confused with one another. However, in the spring of 1973, Michigan Chemical ran out of color-coded bags and used plain, brown, fifty-pound bags to package both PBB and magnesium oxide. In addition, Michigan Chemical made during this period an experimental batch of PBB that had a consistency and color similar to its magnesium oxide product. Normally the color and consistency of the two products were quite different.

On April 30, 1974, an inspector with the Food and Drug Administration, who was in the midst of tracking down the cause of an epidemic of cattle illness, found a half-used bag of the Michigan Chemical product Firemaster

Adapted from Michael R. Reich, "Toxic Politics: A Comparative Study of Public and Private Responses to Chemical Disasters in the United States, Italy and Japan" (Ph.D. dissertation, Yale University, 1982).

FF-1 (the experimental batch) in a Michigan feed mill. It was found in a brown bag whose contents were not clearly labeled. Apparently, the PBB product was being mistakenly used as a feed additive.

Six months prior to that discovery, in September 1973, the cows at Rick Halbert's dairy farm, just north of Battle Creek, Michigan, had developed a set of undiagnosable symptoms. The symptoms were teary eyes, runny noses, loss of appetite, and an economically significant decrease in milk production.

Rick Halbert was unable to diagnose these symptoms by himself, and he called in his veterinarian. The veterinarian was also unable to diagnose the problems. At the time, Halbert thought he might have a feed problem. He even suspected that the problem might involve some kind of mistake concerning the magnesium oxide added to his cattle feed. He suspected the additive because one of his neighbors had once had a feed additive problem.

In the first of many communications with the company from which he bought his feed, Farm Bureau Services, Rick Halbert was told by a company veterinarian that his cattle had an "inappetence problem" that might have been caused by moldy corn. The veterinarian explained that the problem couldn't be related to their feed because there had been no additional complaints about the feed in question.

Veterinarians from the Michigan Department of Agriculture looked for and found no evidence of infectious disease in Halbert's cattle. A dairy nutritionist from Michigan State University could find no obvious problems in Halbert's feed regimen. Despite this lack of diagnostic success, Halbert continued to believe that something was really wrong with his cattle. The dimensions of his cattle problem continued to increase, and Halpert also noticed that the rats and cats had completely disappeared from his farm.

He decided to start his own experiments and found that the cows' symptoms abated somewhat when he stopped giving them their regular feed and switched them to freshly cut green chop and baled hay. The cattle began to eat again and milk production ceased to fall. After a number of other experiments, Halbert changed to a different feed, even though he was not yet convinced that his original feed (#402 pellets) was the problem.

At Halbert's request, the Michigan Department of Agriculture ran tests with #402 pellets on mice. Ten days after the experiment began, all of the mice were dead. A second experiment produced the same results and convinced Halbert that a partial solution to his problem had been found.

When he called the executive vice-president of the feed company to give him the new information, the vice-president suggested that Halbert might have stored the pellets improperly and that the mice trial was inconclusive. He told Halbert that "I can't believe those pellets would be causing any trouble."

Several weeks later at a meeting with the same vice-president and several officials from the feed company, the Halberts agreed to share with the company some of their own information about their cattle. The vice-president still denied that the company's feed was in any way related to the Halberts' problem. He also told Halbert that he was still the only farmer reporting problems with #402 pellets. This was not, however, the case. Three months earlier, another farmer had complained of problems with the same pellets, and one month earlier, Farm Bureau Services had discontinued production of #402 pellets. None of this new information was given to Halbert.

Halbert's problems continued to increase, even though he had removed his cattle from the #402 pellets. Calf mortality rose to five times its normal rate, and this was only part of increasingly common reproductive problems in his herd. In addition, the adult cattle developed new symptoms: drooping ears, dull and coarse coats, missing patches of hair that revealed an abnormal elephantine skin on their faces and necks, and a distortion of hoof shape serious enough to cause problems in locomotion.

The livestock problem also threatened the integrity of the Halbert family. "Rick Halbert became obsessed with the problem, ignoring his wife and three young daughters and became more tense and withdrawn as time passed."[1] One of his farmhands died in a tractor accident. Halbert's father wondered if the accident was somehow related to the feed problem. Halbert's wife began to worry that "the invisible enemy" that was afflicting the cattle herd might also be affecting the health of her family.

Halbert next went to the National Animal Disease Laboratory in Ames, Iowa. The laboratory was unable to find any evidence of the usual mold toxin or chemical contaminants in Halbert's feed. By chance, the gas-liquid chromatography machine used for this analysis was left on for eight hours and "a strange series of peaks" was found, indicating the presence of a foreign substance in the feed. However, the laboratory was unable to identify the contaminant and discontinued work on the problem.

Farm Bureau Services tested the feed for the standard pesticides and found that none of them was present. It concluded that the feed was "wholesome and pure." One month later the company also told Halbert that its own feeding experiment with #402 pellets had shown the feed to be harmless. In fact, three of the four calves in the company's experiment had died. Soon thereafter, the company veterinarian told Halbert that he was still unaware of other farmers with similar problems, even though Halbert himself now knew of two such farmers.

The mystery was solved to some extent in April 1974, when Halbert learned from a private laboratory that bromine had been detected in his feed. Armed with that information and the molecular weights of the peaks from low-resolution mass spectrometry, Halbert was able to locate an analytical chemist at the U.S. Department of Agriculture who identified the contaminant as PBB, a flame retardant manufactured by Michigan Chemical Corporation. Halbert immediately recognized Michigan Chemical as the same company that manufactured the magnesium oxide that Farm Bureau Services adds to their feed.

With Rick Halbert's discovery that his cattle problems were probably the result of a PBB contamination of his feed, a whole new series of uncertainties and conflicts emerged in the Michigan PBB contamination. It turned out that hundreds of Michigan farmers were having the same exact livestock problems as Halbert. A number of public health, political, and legal problems arose as it slowly became evident that a sizable number of Michigan livestock herds had been consuming PBB-contaminated feed for a lengthy period. Attempts to resolve these problems foundered on a whole new group of uncertainties regarding the contamination and its consequences.

Once it had been determined that the Farm Bureau Services had been selling PBB-contaminated feed, the problem entered the public and political arena. Within weeks of the discovery, the U.S. Food and Drug Administration declared that milk and milk products containing more than 1.0 part of PBB per million parts milk should be neither sold nor consumed. At the same time, the Michigan Department of Agriculture ordered seven farms to stop selling milk because PBB contamination of their milk exceeded the FDA guideline. The state also forbade the selling of the contaminated cattle for slaughter for meat. Within three weeks, an additional twenty-three farms had been quarantined by the state.

During this period, the Michigan Department of Agriculture announced that the PBB problem was limited to a "very few" farms and that there was "little need for concern about the public milk supplies." The department also called a meeting in which state policy regarding the PBB contamination was determined. The meeting was chaired by the director of the department. He set the meeting's tone at the outset and expressed his approach to the problem in saying, "I think that milk is a pretty good product and I hope that out of this we don't do anything to injure the dairy industry."

Participants in the meeting eventually put together a public statement about the problem. One of their central concerns in drafting this statement was to understate the problem so as not to "alarm the public." The meeting had received reassurances from Michigan Chemical Corporation and Farm Bureau Services that the contamination was a limited problem and virtually under control.

The original quarantine had brought its share of economic and psychological problems to the farmers with contaminated herds.

> They could not sell the cows or their milk. Neither could they kill the animals, since no burial site existed to dispose of the PBB contaminated carcasses. . . . They continued feeding the cows, dumping the milk, and losing hundreds of dollars a day. . . . [they] had no idea if or when the responsible parties would pay for losses. . . . Each quarantined farmer was watching the death of a herd and business he had worked years to create,

and the death of animals whom he loved like . . . family. Halbert recalled: "I began to understand why people jumped out of windows during the great depression. Suddenly the future appeared so uncertain that it was mind boggling."[2]

By October 1974, 151 farms had been quarantined by the state Department of Agriculture. A total of 6,700 cattle, 341 sheep, and 850,000 chickens were quarantined.

The issue of acceptable levels of PBB contamination for Michigan milk and meat became a central problem in the growing controversy. It turned out to be exceedingly difficult to arrive at a rationally and empirically determined level of acceptable PBB exposure for human beings. The question was essentially this: what levels of PBB contamination in milk, meat, and eggs would not cause untoward effects in human beings?

The original FDA level of one part per million (PPM) was called into question when a number of farmers reported health and milk production problems in livestock that had PBB levels below that threshold. The implication seemed to be that if PBB levels less than the one PPM threshold were causing illness in livestock, they were probably also causing illness in human beings.

As a result, the U.S. Food and Drug Administration lowered its definition of acceptable PBB levels from 1.0 to 0.3 PPM in milk, meat, and poultry and from 1.0 to 0.5 PPM in eggs. In turn, the Michigan Department of Agriculture also adopted these levels and announced that an additional fifty or sixty herds might have to be quarantined.

Soon thereafter, even these new guidelines were called into question. Dairy farmers continued to report serious health problems in cattle that were producing milk with PPB levels below 0.3 PPM. In a survey reported in early 1975, the state of Michigan found that in 286 "low-level herds"—those with detectable PBB levels below 0.3 PPM—about half had health problems similar to those in herds with PBB levels greater than 0.3 PPM.

Nonetheless, the Michigan Department of Agriculture did not lower the level of acceptable PBB contamination. As the contamination began to be front page news, both houses of the Michigan legislature passed a resolution calling on the state to quarantine all livestock showing a detectable PBB level. One week later, a major Michigan supermarket chain announced that it would not sell Michigan products contaminated by PBB. That same day Governor Miliken telephoned the commissioner of the Food and Drug Administration and asked for a public statement of reassurance that Michigan's food products were safe. The FDA issued the requested statement later that same day.

At a hearing on May 29, 1975, the Michigan Department of Agriculture decided to continue to abide by the existing FDA guidelines. In making this decision, it said that, "The decision must be based on either relying on presently available scientific evidence and retaining the present action levels, or deciding in favor of a lower, unsupported action level based on fear of unproven long range health hazards."[3]

The dilemma was genuine. At the time, there were no existing studies of the chronic human health effects of PBB exposure. No one knew what, if any, level of PBB in the human body was safe. The levels that the FDA were using had been extrapolated from studies of the health effect of a related contaminant, polychlorinated biphenyl (PCB). Under these circumstances, the Michigan Department of Agriculture decided to assume that future studies of the health effects of the PBBs would find no problems. It continued to permit the sale of contaminated produce.

The problem presented a moral dilemma for the farmers who owned "low-level herds." One such farmer, who decided on his own to kill his contaminated cattle, said afterwards, "One state inspector told me not to eat the meat and milk from my own cows, but in the next breath he told me I could sell them for the public. That didn't make sense."[4] At public hearings called by a state legislator, another farmer said, "If you think you're a Christian, are you going to ship them and let your neighbors eat them?"[5]

The legislative hearings at which the above testimony was given brought affected farmers together for the first time. As one woman described it, "Until [the hearings] farmers suffered on an individual basis. We had not wanted to talk about our problems. We blamed ourselves. . . . The hearing brought people together. We began to realize that there are others in the same boat."[6]

Undiagnosed health problems among farm families were one of the important subjects of discussion at the hearings. One woman testified, "Well, we all experienced sluggishness, tiredness. We have a boy that's about fifteen that I swear he sleeps more than, you just wouldn't believe a child of that age would sleep almost constantly. He experiences stomach pains, he's lost a lot of school, he's not growing properly for a boy his age according to his doctor. My husband has chest pains. We have a swelling of the joints, he has dizziness, loss of balance."[7]

In March 1976 Governor Miliken created a PBB Scientific Advisory Panel. It issued a report at the end of May that shocked Michigan. The report said, "No significant acute effects of PBB have yet been documented in man" and "no specific disease or symptomatology in animals or man can presently be associated with exposure to low levels of PBB." It went on, "The potential acute and chronic health hazards, the uncertainty in regard to carcinogenicity and teratogenicity, the long-term tissue retention and possible accumulation of PBB, and the present geographical containment of contaminated stock argues for the institution of an action level no higher than that presently found in control populations of animals." The panel unanimously recommended reducing PBB action levels to the minimal detectable limits: 0.005 PPM in meat and 0.001 in milk.[8]

One month later the state agricultural commission, at the recommendation of the director of the Department of Agriculture, decided to retain the existing FDA action levels of 0.3 PPM in both meat and milk. This decision permitted the continued sale of produce from the low-level herds.

The remainder of 1976 saw a succession of studies indicating that the PBB contamination might be affecting human health. At the outset, the authorities thought that the human health effects of the contamination would not be very important. At the Department of Agriculture meeting held in May 1974, it was generally agreed that the problem was a minor livestock problem. However, the Michigan Department of Public Health initiated in that month a preliminary screening study of 211 people who were living on Michigan farms. The department reported that the survey "showed that people were directly exposed to PBB and that the chemical was circulating in their blood. But the department concluded that the study did not reveal 'a medical syndrome, or group of symptoms, which can be related to PBB.'"[9]

This preliminary survey was followed up by a controlled study of 300 people. The findings of this study supported those of the preliminary study. The authors of the study reported that (1) there was no connection between PBB contamination and any human symptoms, (2) trace amounts of PBB found in the blood do not "have any clinical significance," and (3) "so far we have found no real difference in the health status of those exposed and those not exposed, and we have no reason to believe that any will be found."[10]

These conclusions were based on a study completed only months after the contamination had been discovered. It is noteworthy that 70 percent of the subjects in this study's control group were found to have detectable PBB levels in their blood.

The problem of human health effects disappeared, more or less, from the public eye for the two years that followed. It began to reemerge when families from contaminated farms reported at legislative hearings that they were experiencing undiagnosable medical problems. In August 1976 Michigan's Department of Public Health made the serendipitous discovery, as part of a study of pesticide contamination, that twenty-two out of twenty-six samples of human breast milk taken from all over Michigan contained detectable levels of PBB. Of ten samples of breast milk taken from outside of Michigan, not one contained even a trace of PBB.

In announcing the results, the state director of health said, "There is absolutely no evidence to date that PBB in mother's milk causes babies to become ill. On the contrary, babies of such nursing mothers appear to be strong and healthy."[11] In October 1976 the Department of Public Health completed a more reliable study that indicated that 96 percent of the women living in Michigan's lower peninsula had PBB in their breast milk. The highest reported level was 1.2 PPM. Nonetheless, the department said, "The levels of PBB are not sufficient to discourage Michigan mothers from breast feeding if they so desire."[12]

Irving Selikoff, who was already well known for his work on the health effects of asbestos, took a different approach. He came to Michigan in November 1976 at the invitation of Michigan's Speaker of the House. Upon his arrival, he recommended that women avoid breast feeding until it was proven that their milk was free of PBB.

Selikoff came to Michigan with a thirty-five member team and examined 1,000 farm families. The Selikoff team wanted to determine whether or not the people most likely to have high exposures to PBB were having health problems as a result of those exposures.

Selikoff's group immediately found a recurring pattern of undiagnosable symptoms among the exposed families; joint problems, fatigue, dizziness, memory problems, excessive sweating, wounds that wouldn't heal, darkening of the skin, and hypersensitivity to sunlight. However, the team was unable to determine if the symptoms were being caused by PBB exposure.

In a report published in January 1977, Selikoff wrote that his group had found nervous system, musculoskeletal, and gastrointestinal abnormalities. He emphasized that he did not have enough data with which to reach enduring conclusions about the relationship between these symptoms and PBB contamination. Thus the question of the human health effects of the Michigan contamination was left unresolved. Symptomatic families living on contaminated farms remained uncertain about the meaning of those symptoms.

A gubernatorial race was held in Michigan in 1978, and the PBB issue was central in the campaign. The incumbent governor, Miliken, won reelection. Afterwards the PBB issue disappeared, without resolution of many of the issues that the contamination had raised.

7
Love Canal Case Study

The Love Canal accident all began with the entrepreneurial dreams of William T. Love. At the end of the nineteenth century he conceived of a plan to dig a canal that would reroute water from the Niagara River (and in the process bypass Niagara Falls) to generate electricity along the canal. His vision for the canal included building a planned community around the industry that would undoubtedly be attracted to the site because of the inexpensive electricity that would be available there.

The plan actually got off the ground, but it came to an ignominious halt when investors withdrew their capital during the depression of the mid-1890s. Despite the failure of his project, Mr. Love did not fail to leave his mark upon the Niagara Falls area landscape. He left a partially finished canal that measures some three thousand feet long, sixty feet wide, and ten feet deep. All in all, it is quite a monument to his unfulfilled and ambitious vision. That unfinished canal, known as the Love Canal, is now within the city limits of Niagara Falls, N.Y.

In 1942 Hooker Electrochemical Company bought the canal and some adjacent land as a site for the disposal of chemical wastes. It used the site for this purpose between 1942 and 1952. During this period Hooker deposited more than 21,000 tons of chemical waste into the huge trench.

By 1953 the canal was almost full, and Hooker covered it over with earth and clay. The site was reclaimed by grass and weeds, and as time passed it came to look like an innocuous and natural field. The history of the site was more or less concealed by the combined actions of Hooker Chemical and nature.

In 1953 Hooker Chemical sold the site to the school board of Niagara Falls for the token sum of one dollar. The deed of sale included a passage in which the city of Niagara Falls assumed all subsequent liability related to the chemical wastes that had been placed in the canal and stated that no lawsuit could ever be lodged for damages attributed to those wastes.

In 1954 construction of an elementary school was begun on the site. The school opened its doors to students in 1955, and 400 children began to attend

Adapted from Adeline G. Levine, *Love Canal: Science, Politics and People* (Lexington, Mass.: Lexington Books, 1982); Martha R. Fowlkes and P.Y. Miller, "Love Canal: The Social Construction of Disaster" (Submitted to the Federal Emergency Management Agency, October 1982).

school on top of the old dump site. These students, as well as additional children who lived in the surrounding neighborhood, routinely used the grounds adjacent to the school as a playground. The fields on which these children played were also located directly above the now invisible chemical waste dump site.

Eventually a substantial residential community was built on the land adjacent to the school. Approximately 1,000 families ended up living in the immediate area. Most of them had absolutely no idea that they were moving into an area that had recently been an active dump site for toxic chemicals.

Nonetheless, the canal was problematic for the area's residents almost from the beginning. As early as the 1950s, area residents were troubled by the presence of unfamiliar and disturbing chemical odors, particularly after heavy precipitation. These odors were generally dismissed or ignored because residents believed that the odors were coming from nearby chemical plants. However, problems related to the canal were not limited to odors. During the entire thirty-five year period between the covering of the canal and the public emergence of the Love Canal disaster, problems of one sort or another continued to become apparent to the residents of the Love Canal area.

Children playing barefoot near the school developed skin problems on their feet. Neighborhood dogs suffered the same fate: their noses and bellies would become irritated after they ran on the fields covering the old dump site. On numerous occasions, chemical waste products spontaneously appeared on the ground over the canal. Holes would spontaneously appear in playing field surfaces as the rusting fifty-five-gallon waste barrels decayed and collapsed.

Sometimes toxic substances actually made their way into nearby homes. Thick black substances were found on some basement walls and floors. In 1965 one area resident found a black oily substance in a sump pump located in his basement. Spontaneous chemical fires were also reported over the canal, and small explosions were noticed.

During the 1970s the toxic presence of the canal became more evident. Large puddles containing contaminated water appeared in residential backyards after heavy rainstorms and remained there for days. The intensity and frequency of chemical odors increased. Holes appeared in the baseball diamond located on the school grounds.

In spite of these events, most neighborhood residents seem to have felt at the time that the area was safe. The presence of a school built by the city of Niagara Falls and the endowing of mortgages by the Federal Housing Administration seemed to imply that all was well. In addition, there was no direct indication that a health problem was present in the community.

Complaints were made, however, by some of the area's residents. From time to time complaints were lodged with both the city and Hooker Chemical. Typically, these complaints resulted in either an inspection of some sort or in "short term remedial measures."[1] For the most part, it seems that neither area residents nor governmental officials thought of the Love Canal as a health problem of any consequence.

This picture began to change in 1976 when the International Joint Commission—a joint commission of the United States and Canada—detected traces of the insecticide Mirex in Lake Ontario fish. The New York Department of Environmental Conservation traced the Mirex to another Hooker Corporation dump site near the Love Canal.

Several months later a series of articles tracing the history of Love Canal appeared in the Niagara Gazette. The Department of Environmental Conservation inaugurated an investigation of Love Canal, and a chain of events was set off that led to an investigation by several government agencies. The Environmental Protection Agency began in October 1977 to analyze air samples from the basements of Love Canal homes. The Department of Environmental Conservation sampled basement sump pumps, soil, and storm sewers. The New York State Department of Health began to do preliminary studies as well. As evidence built up regarding the environmental contamination of the Love Canal area, the State Department of Health began to conduct a health survey and to take blood samples from area residents.

All of this new activity—the environmental monitoring, the health surveys, and the news media coverage—served notice to Love Canal residents that something might be genuinely wrong with the dump site. Government officials from a number of agencies constantly appeared to measure one thing or another. News stories relating the dangers of the Love Canal began to appear regularly in the media. Surely, the residents began to think, with all of this demonstrated concern, something must truly be wrong. Suddenly the irritated skin, the pernicious odors, the undiagnosed illnesses, and chemical residues began to seem as if they had been, all along, the early signs of an invisible and impending health crisis.

Government officials began to hold public meetings in the spring and summer of 1978 to explain their emerging awareness of the problem to Love Canal residents. For the residents, here was yet another indication that the canal posed a serious threat to their health. Certainly, they reasoned, if officials were going so far as to hold meetings to explain the canal, the situation must be dangerous. They attended these meetings in hope of figuring out exactly what was going on.

What they learned at the public meetings was that information about the canal was abundantly available, but that the information did not help them make personal decisions about the dangers posed by the chemicals leeching out of the Love Canal. For example, at one meeting on July 19, 1978, officials passed out the results of their studies of the presence of chemicals in the basements of Love Canal neighborhood houses. The results were passed out to individual houseowners, and in a large number of cases, the results indicated that several chemicals were present in neighborhood basements. Worried residents wanted to know the meaning of these findings; they wanted to know if the chemicals posed a threat to the health of their families. They were more than a little surprised and alarmed to discover that the answer to that question was not available. The officials present at this meeting were simply unable to tell the residents whether the test results meant that their houses were safe or unsafe. Thus residents were able to ascertain that their housing was contaminated with potentially dangerous chemicals, but they were unable to determine what the existing or future health effects of that contamination would be.

> Residents attended meetings; listened to the statements by officials, who either denied problems existed or pointed with alarm and then offered no help or advice; listened to neighbor's accounts of the meetings; and read the comments about their homes and neighborhood. They became terrified that their homes—especially their basements, where many had innocently built bedrooms and family rooms—were dangerous places. . . . What frightened them even more, however, was the possibility, first, that no one in authority knew what was really wrong, and, second, that even if they did know exactly what was wrong, maybe no one would help anyway.[2]

The problem was brought temporarily into focus when on August 2, 1978, Dr. Robert P. Whalen, the commissioner of health for the state of New York, issued a Health Department order regarding Love Canal. He announced that the "Love Canal chemical waste landfill constitutes a public nuisance and an extremely serious threat and danger to the health, safety and welfare of those using it, living near it or exposed to the conditions emanating from it."[3]

Whalen made seven recommendations, four of which are as follows:

1. All pregnant women living in buildings adjacent to the canal should be temporarily evacuated.
2. All children under two years of age living in buildings adjacent to the canal should be temporarily evacuated.
3. Residents should avoid going into their basements.
4. Residents should avoid eating anything from their gardens.

To be told not to go into your own basement because it might be dangerous is a pretty alarming state of affairs, and now much of the Love Canal neighborhood was certain that something was really wrong. For them, Commissioner Whalen's statement was confirmation that the canal was posing a genuine threat to the health of the surrounding community. However, now the question arose as to what should be done about it. The commissioner's announcement created more uncertainties and problems for the residents than it resolved. This new set of uncertainties was brought into ironically sharp focus by one additional development.

On August 7, 1978, the governor of New York, Hugh Carey, visited the Love Canal neighborhood and announced that the state of New York would be willing to buy all of the homes adjacent to the canal. Some 300 families living in what came to be known as rings I and II were to be permanently relocated. The statement represented a revision of Commissioner Whalen's earlier recommendations.

It must have seemed to Governor Carey that this bold action would be perceived as both generous and effective. However, neither he, his staff, nor his Department of Health seems to have anticipated or understood the effect that the relocation plan would have upon the remaining residents of the Love Canal neighborhood, the residents of the area that came to be known as ring III.

There were an additional 700 families living in ring III housing, many of whom also considered themselves to be at risk from the chemical wastes located in the canal. They had a particularly difficult time understanding how anyone could be so certain that the chemicals escaping from the Love Canal were fastidiously stopping at the boundary between ring II and ring III homes. How, they wanted to know, did the state know that the health effects of the dump site were confined to rings I and II?

It was unclear to the ring III residents how one house in ring II could be endangered, while another house, just across the street in ring III, could be considered to be safe. It was primarily around this issue of boundary that conflict and uncertainty developed in the years that followed New York's decision to purchase those homes closest to the canal. In purchasing the homes in rings I and II, the state had declared an "official perimeter of risk"[4] that did not make sense to the remaining Love Canal residents.

At the time of Governor Carey's and Commissioner Whalen's statements, there had not been any thorough studies of the health effects of the chemicals escaping from the canal. A preliminary study had demonstrated "a slight increase in risk for spontaneous abortion among residents of the canal."[5] The state must have made its decisions on the basis of this one health study and a group of environmental studies that had already been done, that is, on the studies that had demonstrated the contamination of the air, soil, and water of the Love Canal environment.

Thus, in addition to recommending the relocation of residents, Whalen also ordered that extensive studies be undertaken to determine the prevalence of chronic disease among residents living adjacent to the canal. These new studies came to hold a very important place in the minds of the Love Canal residents remaining in ring III. They were led to believe that these new studies would indicate whether the canal had been affecting their health all along and whether they would be able to move from the area with the financial assistance of the state. They were soon disappointed.

It is probably accurate to say that a sizable proportion of the remaining Love Canal residents believed that their situation was already dangerous, and that they were simply waiting for scientific studies that would demonstrate this fact and make it possible for them to leave. The state of New York, on the other hand, seems to have had a somewhat more complicated perspective on the matter. Public and private statements by the governor and the new commissioner of health[6] indicated that the state would not be able to provide the funds to purchase ring III homes and effect a permanent relocation of all Love Canal residents. Nevertheless, a number of state officials were simultaneously seeking funds from the federal government to purchase those homes. They sought these funds on the grounds that the Love Canal threatened the health of ring III residents. At the same time, they were telling ring III residents that studies would have to be done to determine if this was the case.[7]

Thus the state of New York, as well as the Love Canal residents, appears to have been caught in a bind. The state was simultaneously: (1) doing health studies at Love Canal, (2) telling ring III residents that they would not purchase ring III homes because it was safe there, and (3) requesting funds of the federal government with which to relocate ring III residents. The remaining Love Canal residents were trapped on the receiving end of this same bind. They were waiting for the state and the federal government to carry out the studies that would document the danger present in their community but were beginning to suspect that honest studies would never be done.

In the twenty-seven months that followed the announced permanent relocation of ring I and II residents, the state Department of Health publicly announced only two findings from its health studies of the Love Canal residents. These announcements became part of a larger nexus of events that convinced many of the Love Canal residents that every additional moment that they continued to live in their neighborhood was done at great risk to their health. The most prominent occurrences in this two-year train of events were as follows:[8]

1. John Kenny, aged seven, died suddenly in October 1978 amid speculation that his death was linked to exposure to toxic chemical wastes.

2. Local newspapers reported New York State Department of Health identification of radioactivity near the school on 93rd Street in September 1978.

3. The 93rd Street school was subsequently closed in August 1979 following New York State Department of Health notification to the school physician that dioxin had been found in Black Creek, which borders the school grounds.

4. The New York State Department of Health confirmed the presence of chemical leachate (water containing chemicals) in the wider Love Canal area in November 1978.

5. Preliminary results of epidemiological research conducted by Love Canal Homeowners Association consultant Beverly Paigen, Ph.D., appeared in local newspapers in October 1978. Data revealed a significant correlation between a range of self-reported health problems and residential location in the so-called "wet" areas, where homes lie on or near the path of old streambeds that also traverse the canal site.

6. "On February 8, 1979, Dr. [David] Axelrod [the new commissioner of the New York State Department of Health] recommended the temporary relocation of all pregnant women and children under two living in the six block area east of the canal [ring III]." The recommendation was made on the basis of the findings that there was a twofold increase in the wet area of rates of miscarriage, fetal malformation, and infants with low birth weights.[9]

7. In December 1978 the New York State Department of Health confirmed the presence of dioxin in soil samples taken from 93rd Street.

8. Results of tests indicating abnormal liver function in some area residents were released to the public by the State Department of Health in November 1978.

9. The chromosome study sponsored by the U.S. Environmental Protection Agency was publicized in May 1980. It revealed an apparent elevation in the incidence of chromosome damage among Love Canal residents.

Each of these public scientific events suggested to neighborhood residents that their situation was indeed dangerous. Their dilemma was this: they had become convinced that the area was dangerous and that they should be relocated, and yet, government officials were holding that the danger was uncertain because there were not yet any conclusive studies documenting the health effects of the chemicals located in the canal. As a result, angry and disrespectful meetings occurred between Love Canal residents and state officials. Many residents thought that under the circumstances it was inhumane for the state to keep them in the area until definitive scientific confirmation was available.

The lid finally came off of the pot with the results of the EPA chromosome study. The announcement caused panic and fear in the streets of the Love Canal neighborhood. When the White House announced, three days after the results of the EPA study had been made public, that it would not support the relocation of ring III residents, two EPA officials were detained and held hostage for six hours at the Love Canal Homeowners Association office. The next day the White House announced that money would be made available to permit temporary evacuation of the 700 remaining families.

Another consequence of the chromosome study was that neighborhood residents began to make significant personal decisions. The EPA had sent a group of physicians, scientists, and lawyers to explain the results of the study to its subjects. As a result, the study was received by neighborhood residents hungry for facts as credible information on which significant decisions could be made.

For example, one man who was found to have chromosomal damage called his twenty-seven-year-old daughter to let her know that she and her husband should seriously reconsider their week-old decision to have children. "By the time we finished talking her voice was so low—I think she was almost crying."[10] Another woman made the decision to have her fallopian tubes tied.[11]

Yet even the chromosome study was to become a source of uncertainty for the Love Canal residents. In yet another twist, the validity of this study came under immediate and vicious attack from a variety of sources. As a result, not even this study was to remain a firm piece of cognitive ground on which Love Canal residents could stand and make decisions about real and significant issues in their lives. The chromosome study, which had been presented at EPA news conferences as a significant finding regarding the health effects of the canal, had only been a pilot study of thirty-six subjects. As such, it was a vulnerable study and within weeks its validity had disappeared in a swarm of both negative and positive reviews.

As a result, the situation did not resolve with either the chromosome study or with the White House announcement that temporary relocation of ring III residents would be financed by the federal government. Residents were soon told that permanent relocation could be contingent on the results of further studies. Then the EPA reversed itself and decided that although it would fund further Love Canal studies, it would not use the results of the studies to make any recommendations regarding the relocation issue or any policy decisions regarding the Love Canal. The Love Canal Homeowners Association responded to this decision by refusing to participate in any further studies unless they were allowed to participate in the design and execution of those studies.

A summer of feverish work eventually led to an agreement in August 1980 that provided money for the purchase of the remaining Love Canal homes. As of October 1982, 402 of the 550 ring III houses had been purchased by the Love Canal Revitalization Agency—the agency set up to buy the housing. This "second relocation was construed as a mental health rather than a physical health emergency."[12] That is, it was not based on any estimation of the somatic health effects of the canal.

It now appears that definitive information of the health effects of the canal on area residents will not be forthcoming. On April 1, 1981, the Reagan administration canceled all of the proposed studies of the health effects of the Love Canal toxic waste dump site.

8
Atomic Veteran Case Study

The subject of this case study, Ted Miller, enlisted in the U.S. Navy in 1938 and was honorably discharged in 1947. He fought in the Pacific theater during World War II and passed through Hiroshima the day after V-J Day. In 1946 Ted's ship was assigned to participate in Operation Crossroads—the first post–World War II nuclear weapons test performed by the United States. Operation Crossroads consisted of two tests code-named Able and Baker. Both of these test bombs were detonated at the Bikini Atoll in the summer of 1946. Ted participated in both of them.

During both detonations, Ted stood on the deck of his ship and watched the bombs explode. He estimated that during both tests his ship was located about six to ten miles from the site of the explosion. He reported that neither he nor his crewmates wore protective clothing or glasses during either test. He did not cover his eyes, and he actually looked in the direction of the blast as he had been ordered to do.

At the time of the tests, Ted felt absolutely certain that he was safe. That is, he believed that the radiation released by the bombs posed no threat to his health. He held this belief because he and his shipmates had been told by the navy that it was safe. It had never occurred to him to question the information that he had received. In his own words, "none of us thought it was dangerous."

However, as the years passed, he changed his mind. He was quite emphatic before his death in stating that he believed that his posttest medical problems had been caused by the radiation to which he was exposed at Bikini.

On the occasion of both tests, Ted's ship steamed back into Bikini Lagoon, where the bombs had been detonated, just two hours after the explosion. After the Able test, Ted actually lived on a target ship (the *U.S.S. Dawson*) in Bikini Lagoon for three weeks (July 2 to July 24). During the Able test, the *Dawson* had been left in the lagoon near the site where the bomb was detonated. During the three weeks after the explosion, Ted and his shipmates "kept up the normal ship routine and checked the ship for damage." They also drank desalinated water from the lagoon.

On July 25, 1946, Ted reboarded his original ship and left the lagoon to watch the second test. The circumstances were the same as those that prevailed during the first test. Upon returning to the lagoon after the Baker test, he was informed that the *Dawson,* which had been left again in the lagoon, was now too contaminated to permit a crew to live on board. Ted continued to live aboard his original ship in the lagoon until the end of August. However, during August he did board the *Dawson* three times to inspect it for damage.

Ted said that at the time he was not concerned by the fact that the *Dawson* had been declared uninhabitable. He said that he "just didn't know what was going on." In retrospect, however, he thought, "I must have had a feeling," because he remembered that on one occasion, when he was assigned the task of using an acetylene torch to burn radioactive material off the surface of the ship, he would not allow anyone else to do the same task.

Ted remained at Bikini until the end of August 1946 and then was shipped back to San Francisco. He stayed in the navy one more year, and then he began civilian life as a furniture salesman in Ohio. Eventually, he took a job as a civilian employee of the air force. Between 1947 and 1959 Ted said that it never occurred to him that his participation in the bomb tests had endangered his health.

In 1959 he was diagnosed as having cataracts by an air force physician. The same physician told him that his cataracts had been caused by radiation from the bomb tests. By that time it had been discovered that ionizing radiation can cause posterior subcapsular cataracts. One of the first reports published by the Atomic Bomb Casualty Commission was a paper reporting the existence of "Atomic Bomb Cataracts" in both the Hiroshima and Nagasaki populations.

Being a veteran, Ted went to a Veterans Administration hospital to get medical care and compensation for his condition. The Veterans Administration told Ted that his cataracts were unrelated to radiation and that it was "nonsense" to think that they were related. As a result, Ted dropped the idea that his cataracts had been caused by radiation, and he didn't think about the radiation again for several more years.

He said that he felt no need to question the Veterans Administration assessment of the etiology of his cataracts. The idea that radiation had caused his cataracts "sounded fantastic to me. I didn't think the navy would do something like that; that they would expose people like that. It wasn't war."

Over the next two decades Ted's health progressively deteriorated. He developed a number of serious health problems, but the central and most debilitating of these was a chronic respiratory illness of unknown etiology. In February 1960 he developed shortness of breath for the first time. By January 1970 he was diagnosed as having pulmonary insufficiency of unknown etiology. In March 1976 pulmonary function tests demonstrated that he had only 28 percent of his normal respiratory capacity.

Over the years Ted's respiratory condition was the subject of extensive clinical evaluation. However, the cause of this condition remained unknown to both him and his physicians at the time of his death. Several physicians told Ted that he had pneumosclerosis of unknown etiology. Ted reported that in 1980 one of his physicians ventured to tell him that his respiratory problems had probably been caused by radiation.

Ted's health problems were not confined to his eyes and lungs. In 1959 several of the teeth in his upper jaw turned black and brittle and had to be extracted. Again, neither Ted nor his physicians were ever able to determine why his teeth had gone bad.

Ted was also found to have a calcium deposit in his left shoulder and a chronic tendonitis of the neck. He experienced a chronic and undiagnosed pain in his entire right arm and had an undiagnosed growth on the little finger of the same arm.

In addition, Ted and his wife also had severe reproductive problems. Between 1956 and 1963 his wife had four miscarriages. Of the pregnancies that came to term, two of their children were born with severe birth defects. One son was diagnosed as having Down's Syndrome, and a second son was born with what Ted called a "mental condition." The second son has lived most of his life in a California state hospital.

Through almost the entire course of his medical problems, Ted never thought that they were related to the radiation from the bomb tests in which he participated. After all, he reasoned, he had been told by the navy that it was safe. In 1978 he began to reconsider this conclusion when he became aware of a Department of Defense announcement requesting that atomic veterans call a toll-free number in Washington, D.C.

The announcement said that the Department of Defense was attempting to determine if any of the atomic veterans were having radiation-related health problems. The announcement had a profound effect on Ted; causing him to wonder if his and his family's health problems were somehow related to his exposure to radiation. In his own words, "I got to thinking about all of my past sicknesses and realized that none of it had ever made much sense to me."

At the time of the interviews from which this case study is drawn, and later at the time of his death, Ted had a curious, if not paradoxical, attitude about the causes of his medical problems. On the one hand, he felt certain that radiation was the cause of at least some of his problems. On the other hand, he felt a definite sense of loyalty and allegiance to the navy and the country that would not allow him to conclude firmly that radiation was at the heart of the matter. Asked if radiation had been the cause of his undiagnosed illnesses, he once said, "I really wouldn't have the faintest idea if radiation caused these things." On a different occasion, he said that he was convinced that his problems had been caused by the radiation because he had "met so many atomic veterans who have had the same problems."

When asked what his feelings were for the navy, given that radiation might have caused his health problems, Ted said, "I'm more hurt than anything else. They just told us what to do. Who would have ever thought they'd do that to us? I've been disillusioned ever since I found out that people got crippled out there."

Nonetheless, even up to his death, Ted did not hold the navy responsible for the radiological contamination of the sailors who had participated in Operation Crossroads. He thought it must have been "the politicians" who were to blame. He said that he would serve again in the navy without hesitation, but that he would not have participated in the bomb tests if he had understood radiation and would not participate in them in the future. He thinks that "it was wrong" to have soldiers participate in the tests because "you shouldn't expose anyone unnecessarily." His attitude toward the government was changed somewhat by the discovery that he and his fellow sailors might have been exposed to dangerous amounts of radiation as participants in the bomb tests. Ted said, "I don't trust politicians anymore."

There were times when Ted permitted his disillusionment with the navy to reach the point of anger. He said once, "I'm interested in proving that the navy is a liar. They say I didn't stay in the lagoon after the tests, and they say I wasn't contaminated. They hurt a lot of good people out there."

Once Ted realized that radiation may have been the cause of his health problems, he began to accumulate information about all aspects of the exposure of soldiers to radiation. He believed that "if it comes out into the open, all of the people exposed to radiation will get some kind of settlement; and some of them sure need it." He said, however, that "it is more important to prove that the navy lied about radiation than it is to get benefits."

However, several of his experiences with the navy, the Veterans Administration, and private and government physicians left Ted with the feeling that somehow the information that he needed to establish that his or anyone else's illnesses were caused by radiation was not going to be available. When he tried to obtain records to document his exposure to radiation, the navy claimed that he had not lived in Bikini Lagoon during the summer of 1946. They also contended that he had not been exposed to a dangerous amount of radiation at Bikini. The Veterans Administration told him that none of his illnesses were related to radiation and rejected several claims for service-connected medical care and compensation.

He eventually stopped going to the Veterans Administration hospitals because "if I went in and asked for a radiation exam I knew what I'd get. I'd get rejected." In March 1980 Ted received from the Veterans Administration his final rejection for his application for service-connected benefits for his cataracts.

He believed that the VA doctors "get brain washed. They do what their chief tells them. They should have been able to tell me what was wrong with my eyes, but they didn't because they were covering for the government."

His private physicians were equally unable to diagnose or treat his medical problems. He was never able to obtain an explanation for his cataracts, pneumosclerosis, dental problems, shoulder and arm pain, shoulder calcification, cervical tendonitis, and reproductive problems. He saw no signs of coverup in their inability to help him but believed "they just don't understand my situation because they haven't been educated in it."

The last twenty years of Ted's life were years of virtual inactivity. He was unable to work, and he spent most of his time at home listening to music and educational tapes. Even working in the garden was difficult because his respiratory status made walking even a few steps an exhausting task.

In 1978, with his awareness that radiation could have caused his health problems, he began with his wife's assistance to spend four to five hours a day researching radiation and the atmospheric nuclear test in which he participated. He believed, "If I can help prove that they've lied, it will help out the younger atomic veterans."

For the most part Ted kept his concerns and beliefs about radiation private. In his own words, "I don't advertise it. It wouldn't do any good anyway. People are indifferent. They think it's all in my imagination. The whole public feels this way. They don't believe radiation is dangerous or that it has caused atomic veterans to be sick."

Ted died in 1983 of complications of his pulmonary disease. When asked what he wanted most for the atomic veterans, he responded, "to get just compensation and to be understood by doctors."

9
Uncertainty

T he case histories give us some idea of the uncertainties that a person exposed to an invisible environmental contaminant can experience. These uncertainties are about the meaning of various aspects of an invisible exposure, and they result in further uncertainty as to how a person might best respond or adapt to such an exposure. In other words, they generate adaptational dilemmas.

The uncertainty surrounding an invisible exposure is a consequence of the environmental and medical invisibility of the contaminants, and it is a constant and perplexing feature of these exposures. Several investigators have found ambiguity and uncertainty to be central aspects of the circumstances created by an invisible exposure. Michael Reich, for example, in a comparative analysis of three accidents involving toxic chemicals, found that "toxic contamination is an insidious process, not immediately obvious to its victims or others. Toxic effects on humans, animals, and the environment are often ambiguous and difficult to trace back to the causative substance. The nature of toxic contamination, then, makes it difficult for victims to recognize their private trouble as a common plight, due to the invisibility of the toxic agent; the non-specificity of most toxic symptoms; the difficulties of identification of the causative substance; and the geographical distribution of victims."[1] In this passage, Reich refers to three forms of experienced uncertainty: exposure uncertainty, etiological uncertainty, and diagnostic uncertainty. To date, twelve types of uncertainty that can be experienced as a consequence of an invisible exposure have been delineated. A comprehensive typology of all of these experienced uncertainties, as well as their definitions, is presented in this chapter.

Fowlkes and Miller have also taken note of the role of uncertainties in an invisible exposure. They found it instructive to compare the circumstances of a disaster involving toxic chemicals to the circumstances created by a natural disaster:

> In important respects, the situation at Love Canal did not present itself with the clarity that attends natural disasters. That there were chemicals with

known toxic effects to humans present in the landfill is undeniable. That they had made their way to the surface of the landfill in places is undeniable. That the presence of toxic chemicals was confirmed in and/or on the property of some specific landowners is undeniable as well. . . . [However] that the conditions at Love Canal had physically harmed or injured residents, or placed them at widespread risk of physical harm or injury was uncertain from the beginning.[2]

Adeline Levine has also taken note of the multiple uncertainties experienced by the residents of Love Canal as that situation unfolded. She provides a graphic description of the effects of those uncertainties:

At the time that the research reported here began, the stress situation was one where the unexpected "crisis" of learning about the threat had passed and the period of "attrition" resulting from "cumulative exposure to a threat" was in process. Lang and Lang (1964) have described this period as particularly demoralizing, with "the worst kind of threat [being] . . . the generalized dread of the unknown." (pg. 71) At Love Canal, by mid-October of 1978, many people felt they had lost control of major aspects of their lives. They were faced with a hazard of unknown dimensions, with potentially serious consequences for health and financial futures; they felt pressed to make crucial decisions based on little exact information; they were unsure about how to anticipate the future, and they felt that they had little credible authoritative guidance to help them. Whatever tangible support they had received from the government was limited, insufficient and no longer forthcoming.[3]

Levine points out that the uncertainties generated by the Love Canal exposure had further consequences for the Love Canal residents: the uncertainty left them scared and unclear as to how they should respond to the dangers posed by the canal.

Uncertainty is also a central aspect of the experience of being exposed to radiation. Military veterans exposed to ionizing radiation found themselves immersed in a compelling mystery concerning the state of their health. These men were characteristically unable to obtain answers to a number of important questions about their health. Most prominent among these unanswered concerns were questions about the etiology, treatment, and prognosis of their medical problems.[4]

Baum et al. in their study of the psychological effects of the Three Mile Island accident found that the engineering and radiological uncertainties of that accident amplified the perception of threat in the population contending with the health effects of that accident.[5] They found that "the actual dangers posed by the accident, coupled with the fact that nuclear power was involved, were sufficient to evoke concern. Compounding this problem, however, was the information crisis, generating uncertainty about the state of the reactor, the degree of danger present and so on. These uncertainties increased fears, many of which were confirmed by the evacuation advisory. Thus, threat was nurtured in an information vacuum [little believable or consistent information was available] and increased perceptions of threat." This finding is consistent with Janis's ambiguity hypothesis, which holds that ambiguous information about a moderately or severely threatening event will increase the amount of vigilance directed toward that event.

It also appears that the uncertainty encountered as a consequence of an invisible exposure is a painful and fear-producing experience for the exposed person. As noted by Lang and Lang, "the worst kind of threat . . . [is] the dread of the unknown."[6] People exposed to an invisible contaminant often find the resulting uncertainty intolerable. Chicago factory workers suffering from the effects of an undiagnosed carbon monoxide contamination became frantic in their attempts to find the cause of their problem. In the words of one worker, "I got almost hysterical when I couldn't put my finger on what it was." Military participants in nuclear weapons tests developed an active distaste for the uncertainty generated by their exposures to radiation. This intolerance of uncertainty is explained in the following dialogue with an atomic veteran:

> —*How has exposure to radiation changed your life?*
> —I am becoming more and more concerned about my health; my health is slowing me down. It keeps me from planning anything. It has instilled a fear of illness in me. Everytime I get a new symptom, I think it's the end.
> —*How does that affect your life?*
> —It's a fear of the unknown. And it's constant.[7]

Another atomic veteran went so far as to say that "to get a bad diagnosis is better than receiving no diagnosis at all. Otherwise, you keep wondering about it."[8] Hudson found much the same response among people relating to other forms of uncertain threat. They told him that "the worst would be better than this [uncertainty]."[9] Uncertainty in the face of threat generates fear because it makes mastery of that threat a virtually impossible task.

The Typology of Uncertainty

Several forms of uncertainty can be experienced in consequence of an invisible exposure. Describing and defining each of these forms will give us a more precise and empathic understanding of the profound sense of uncertainty that a person can experience as the result of an invisible exposure. The types of uncertainty that can be experienced in consequence of an invisible exposure are listed on page 31. Definitions and examples of each type of uncertainty are given below.

Previous Exposure Uncertainty

Previous exposure uncertainty is uncertainty as to whether one has been exposed to an invisible contaminant in the past. This is actually a question about whether or not one's body has absorbed a dose of an invisible contaminant. In other words, a distinction can be made between being in the presence of an invisible contaminant, on the one hand, and actually absorbing a dose of that contaminant, on the other. For example, a ten-year resident of the Love Canal neighborhood discovers in 1978 that chemicals from the Love Canal toxic waste dump site have been seeping into the environment in which he lives. Despite this belated discovery, the question still remains as to whether or not he has actually absorbed any of those toxic chemicals as a result of living in their presence.

Previous exposure uncertainty can also occur in radiation exposures. A person exposed to nonbackground ionizing radiation is not certain, even if he or she is wearing a dosimeter, whether he or she has actually absorbed any radiation. Exposure to ionizing radiation can be understood as being similar to being caught in a hail of bullets. You may or may not be hit.

Present Exposure Uncertainty

Present exposure uncertainty is uncertainty about whether one is currently in the process of absorbing an invisible contaminant. It involves the same distinction between exposure and absorption discussed above in relation to previous exposure uncertainty. For the Love Canal resident who is now aware of the environmental spread of the chemical wastes placed in the canal, the question becomes: am I now absorbing chemicals from the canal as I stand in my living room or in my garden? Even if the air measurements done in the basement of that person's house reveal the presence of toxic chemicals, it is still unclear whether the residents of that home are actually absorbing those chemicals; which means that there is also uncertainty as to whether evacuation of the house or neighborhood is advisable. Beyond these questions lies the further question of whether an absorbed dose of one of those chemicals will cause the development of a clinically detectable disease.

Evacuation Uncertainty

Evacuation uncertainty is uncertainty as to whether one should leave the geographic or physical locale in which an invisible exposure is occurring. For example, should an entire family evacuate the Three Mile Island area on the third day of a nuclear power plant accident there? Should a family leave the Love Canal neighborhood and buy a new house outside of the area? Should people continue to work at a job in which they are continually being exposed to toxic chemicals?

Evacuation uncertainty is a direct consequence of the exposure and dose uncertainties that attend invisible exposures. If you don't know whether you are actually absorbing an invisible contaminant, how large a dose you are absorbing, or how large a dose is safe, it is difficult if not impossible to evaluate empirically the advisability of evacuating the scene of an exposure. Under such circumstances, an appealing strategy is to preemptively evacuate the situation as a means of precluding further exposure. However, evacuation is a complicated option that can involve selling one's home, losing one's job, or leaving the community in which one has lived an entire life.

Boundary Uncertainty

Boundary uncertainty is uncertainty as to the geographical limits of a dangerous invisible exposure. The issue has arisen primarily when a governmental institution declares that within a certain boundary, conditions are dangerous; but beyond that boundary, conditions are safe. For example, at the time of the Three Mile Island accident, the governor of Pennsylvania ordered an evacuation of pregnant women and children under two years of age who were living within five miles of the power plant. Residents living beyond this boundary were more than a little concerned about how the governor knew that radiological dangers posed by the accident ended abruptly at the five-mile boundary.

As time passed, this boundary took on legal importance. Among other ramifications were compensation for evacuation expenses and financial losses, given only to Three Mile Island area residents living at the time of the accident within the five-mile limit. There was much uncertainty and cynical speculation among area residents as to how the authorities ascertained "that the radiation knew to stop right at the five-mile mark."[10]

Similar boundary uncertainty arose at Love Canal. The state of New York originally decided to purchase homes in rings I and II of the Love Canal neighborhood. They announced that it was dangerous in those areas, but not in ring III. Again, the residents of ring III housing wanted to know exactly how the state knew that the chemical leachates were stopping at the boundary of ring III. Why, they wanted to know, was the house in ring II dangerous, but the house across the street in ring III safe? This boundary distinction was of great importance because it determined which houses were bought by the state.

Dose Uncertainty

Dose uncertainty is uncertainty as to how large a dose a person has absorbed of an invisible contaminant. Most often, it is not possible to quantify the absorbed dose of an invisible contaminant. Dose uncertainty may occur for any number of reasons. Often it occurs because no one was aware at the time of exposure that an exposure was occurring. For example, toxic exposures at Love Canal probably went on for years before they were finally discovered in 1978. The majority of radiation released at the Three Mile Island accident was released during the first two days of the accident—long before area residents evacuated or understood that radiation releases were happening.

Dose uncertainty can also occur during a known exposure when monitoring of that exposure is not carried out. Three Mile Island is a good example of this type of circumstance, as is the dioxin contamination that occurred at Seveso, Italy. Both adequate population monitoring and monitoring of individual doses were nonexistent at these accidents. The logistics of such an exercise would have been awesome, expensive, and impossible.

Finally, dose uncertainty can occur because the technology needed to measure a particular type of exposure has not been developed. The situation of the atomic veterans who participated in atmospheric nuclear weapons tests is a good example of this circumstance. At the time of their test involvement, radiation dosimetry was still relatively primitive, and accurate measurement of the various fractions of their doses was not possible. In addition, less than half of those men actually wore dosimeters during the tests.[11]

Exposed people want to know their dose for a number of reasons. Probably the most important is that knowing the dose gives people some idea of whether they have been exposed to a dangerous amount of the contaminant. Knowledge of dose is also important if the exposed person wants to file for workers' compensation or take legal action as a consequence of an invisible exposure.

Significance-of-Dose Uncertainty

This form of uncertainty is the uncertainty that occurs when a person knows the amount of the exposure, or dose, to an invisible contaminant, but is unable to ascertain whether such a dose will result in the eventual contraction of contaminant-caused disease. At Love Canal, state health officials were able to give residents measurements of toxic chemical levels in their basements, but were unable to tell the residents the medical significance of those measurements. Atomic veterans who received radiation doses from the Department of Defense were generally unable to find out from their physicians the likely medical consequences of their exposures. In this situation, significance-of-dose uncertainty was further complicated by dose uncertainty.

Latency Uncertainty

Latency uncertainty is perhaps the most disconcerting of the uncertainties experienced by the person exposed to an invisible contaminant. It occurs as a result of an exposure to an invisible contaminant for which there is a latency period between exposure and the time at which any resultant disease might become apparent. It is the experience of knowing that you have been exposed to an invisible contaminant, but of not knowing whether that exposure has already caused biological damage that will result in the appearance of contaminant-caused disease in the future.

Latency is a consequence of the biology of the delayed-onset lesions caused by an invisible contaminant. As discussed in chapter 3, the original somatic lesion caused by radiation is subcellular and does not become apparent for years. People exposed to invisible contaminants can be acutely and painfully aware of this biology of the delayed-onset lesions and can expend a great deal of energy worrying about whether or not they have already been physically injured by an invisible contamination.

Etiological Uncertainty

Etiological uncertainty is uncertainty as to whether or not a given illness has been caused by a previous invisible exposure. It occurs as a consequence of the absence of markers by which the cause of a particular case of a disease can be determined. This is the case, for example, with radiation. Again, there is abundant epidemiological proof that radiation causes several forms of leukemia. Nonetheless, there is no scientific means of determining whether or not a particular case of leukemia has been caused by radiation exposure.

Etiological uncertainty is a recurring and constant feature of the invisible exposures. Yet another example is that it was not possible to determine whether or not the chloracne seen at Seveso or in consequence of the PCB contamination of cooking oil in Japan was caused by the contaminant in question. Nor was it possible to definitively prove that the illness suffered by Michigan livestock herds was caused by the PBB found in their feed. The same type of empirical dilemma also occurred at Three Mile Island and Love Canal.[12]

Ascertaining the etiology of a postexposure illness can become exceedingly important to exposed persons. First, it can provide them with the all important knowledge of why they got sick. Second, it tells them who is responsible for their illness and whether they have been victimized by another human being. Third, it can potentially provide them with an indication of whether someone else should rightly take financial responsibility for their illness.

Nelkin and Brown have noted the importance for exposed workers of knowing the causes of illness that may be related to their occupational exposures to invisible contaminants.

> People who experience illness want to know its cause. They search for causes for practical reasons—to get compensation or to protect their future self. They also feel a personal need to know, a need to define the origins of their problems, to identify a source. Establishing cause is a comment on the social system, a way to define responsibility and to assert control. However, technical uncertainties create problems for workers who want to document their experiences. They are often unable to gain access to the data necessary to evaluate hazards; they find it difficult to isolate cause and effect even when they suspect the workplace is the source of their problems. And they also find it difficult to convince others of the validity of complaints that are not fully supported by the scientific literature. This restricts their ability to make decisions about continuing work, to substantiate requests for better working conditions, and to document their compensation claims.[13]

Diagnostic Uncertainty

Diagnostic uncertainty is uncertainty about the diagnosis of somatic symptoms that become apparent after an invisible exposure. For a variety of reasons that have yet to be sorted out, individuals exposed to the invisible environmental contaminants tend to develop somatic symptoms that their physicians are unable to diagnose. The result is that the exposed persons do not obtain diagnosis or treatment for their symptoms. This predicament is a source of considerable distress for the exposed persons. For them, it means that something is wrong with their bodies, but that they are unable to determine what it is or how to stop it.

This phenomenon has been a central problem for atomic veterans,[14] Love Canal area residents,[15] workers occupationally exposed to toxic chemicals,[16] and owners of livestock exposed to the PBBs.[17] Theoretically, there are three possible explanations for the undiagnosable somatic symptoms seen in people and livestock exposed to invisible contaminants. Either the symptoms are: (1) hypochondriacal, (2) psychosomatic, or (3) the symptoms of a contaminant-caused disease entity that has not yet been recognized by medical science.

Prognostic Uncertainty

Prognostic uncertainty is the uncertainty that people experience about the future of their health after they have come to believe or empirically know that they have been physically harmed by an invisible contaminant. The question that looms before such people is whether or not in the future they will develop contaminant-caused illnesses that will either kill them or seriously compromise the quality of their lives. They most often find that their physicians are unable to answer the question, because the involved contaminants can produce lesions that are invisible during the early period of their existence. Physicians are also unable to empirically resolve the latency uncertainty on which prognostic uncertainty is based.

Treatment Uncertainty

Treatment uncertainty is uncertainty about how to treat a person's symptoms medically. It is a particularly prominent issue for people with undiagnosable symptoms. It was a problem for atomic veterans, when they were told that their undiagnosable symptoms were "all in your head," that is, that these symptoms had a hypochondriacal origin, and that no treatment was necessary.

Coping Uncertainty

Coping uncertainty is uncertainty about how to adapt to an invisible exposure. Evacuation and treatment uncertainties, as discussed above, are forms of coping uncertainty. However, innumerable additional forms of coping uncertainty can and do appear in the course of adapting to an invisible exposure. For example, a woman of childbearing age who has been a long-time resident of the Love Canal neighborhood might be uncertain as to whether she should have her fallopian tubes tied. A dairy farmer might be uncertain as to whether to change feed or to kill his herd. The residents of Seveso, Italy, were uncertain as to the wisdom of returning to their homes after the dioxin contamination that occurred there. The Michigan state government was uncertain as to whether it would be prudent to permit the continued sale and consumption of PBB-contaminated meat, milk, and eggs. Any number of important and concrete coping decisions may become matters of uncertainty because some of the significant information needed to make those decisions is not available.

Financial Uncertainty

Financial uncertainty is uncertainty as to who is morally responsible for the financial costs and losses incurred as a result of an invisible exposure. Who will pay for the necessary medical care? Who will pay for the damage done to a person's life? And who will pay for the care of children with birth defects? It is also uncertain whether or not one will be able to afford the financial costs of an exposure, if no one is going to help.

Financial uncertainty is a direct consequence of etiological uncertainty. If it is impossible to determine whether a given invisible exposure has caused a particular case of an illness, then it will be almost impossible to decide who is financially responsible for the illnesses suffered by an individual who has been exposed to an invisible contaminant. Again, this form of uncertainty is laden with exceedingly tangible and important life consequences for the exposed person. One example is the Love Canal resident who can not afford to move from his home unless it is scientifically proven that the canal has been causing significant illness among area residents. Only then will the state purchase area housing and make the move financially possible.

The Veterans Administration will not give medical care and compensation to an atomic veteran unless it can be empirically proven that his illness has been caused by radiation. The Veterans Administration holds to this position even though they know that it is scientifically impossible to adduce such proof for any radiogenic lesion. The Michigan dairy farmer will not be compensated for the loss of his herd and business unless it can be proven that his herd's illness has been caused by PBBs.

Conclusion

The most immediate consequences of the uncertainty caused by an invisible exposure are fear and a very literal inability to cope with or adapt to the health threats posed by an invisible contamination. Coping with any threatening situation is both mediated by and requires the cognitive appraisal of that situation. The cognitive appraisal of threat requires the availability of information about the threat in question. The issue at which we will look in the next several chapters is this: How does the appraisal of and the adaptation to an invisible exposure proceed, if the information needed to make that appraisal and adaptation is not available?

10
Stress Theory

Exposure to ionizing radiation poses a threat to the health and safety of human beings. Ionizing radiation, which is the type of radiation released from nuclear weapons and nuclear power plants, is a generic term for several forms of radiation. Each type of ionizing radiation (for example, gamma rays, x-rays, and neutrons) can damage biological tissue because it ionizes the atoms present in that tissue. Ionization changes the structure of the molecules in which the ionized atoms are located, and the result can be a molecular lesion that eventually becomes a detectable illness. For example, if ionizing radiation strikes and ionizes one of the many atoms located in a DNA molecule, the result is a genetic mutation. This mutation can become, over time, a cancer or a birth defect.

As a result of its ability to ionize atoms anywhere in the body, ionizing radiation can cause a wide spectrum of clinical illness. Radiogenic illness falls basically into two broad categories: acute radiation sickness and delayed radiation illness (DRI). Acute radiation sickness is an acute illness whose symptoms become manifest within days of an exposure to a large dose of radiation. It appears that a dose of one hundred rads is the approximate minimum dose that can produce the symptoms of acute radiation sickness.[1] In the course of a chest x-ray, a person is exposed to approximately 0.01 rads of ionizing radiation.[2] The LD-50, the dose at which 50 percent of exposed persons will die of acute radiation sickness, is something on the order of 400 rads.[3]

The symptoms of acute radiation sickness vary with dose but can include intractable nausea, vomiting, and diarrhea leading to profound dehydration; thrombocytopenia and the resultant tendency to hemorrhage; decreased resistence to infection as a result of radiogenic bone marrow destruction; and tremors, convulsions, ataxia, and death.[4] Acute radiation sickness is still a relatively rare phenomenon. One must absorb a large dose of radiation to develop this illness. To the best of our knowledge, there have been only a handful of occasions upon which large numbers of people have developed acute radiation sickness: the World War II bombings of Hiroshima and Nagasaki and the recent nuclear power plant accident at Chernobyl are examples. There is some evidence to suggest that a fourth probable occasion was the nuclear accident that occurred at a nuclear waste dump site in the Ural Mountains of the Soviet Union in 1965.

Exposure to ionizing radiation can also cause a large spectrum of delayed radiation illnesses. The most widely recognized forms of delayed radiation illness are those caused by radiation damage to chromosomes: the radiogenic cancers and birth defects. A chromosome is a single strand of DNA, and a chromosomal mutation is an alteration in the base sequence of that DNA molecule. Cancers are a consequence of chromosomal mutations in somatic cells, and birth defects are a consequence of chromosomal mutations in germ, or reproductive, cells.

It is less well known that radiation can also cause illness as a consequence of radiogenic damage to the nonchromosomal elements of animal cells. Radiation can cause cytoplasmic damage, and in so doing cause a number of nontumorous forms of delayed radiation illness. The Soviet literature recognizes three broad, pathologically defined categories of nontumorous DRI:[5]

1. *Aplastic or hypoplastic disease:* Illness caused by a decreased or absent cell population in a particular anatomical location as a consequence of radiogenic cell death.
2. *Sclerotic disease.* Illness caused by the presence of scar tissue in a particular anatomical location as a consequence of radiogenic cell death.
3. *Dyshormonal disease:* Illness characterized by an endocrine imbalance as a consequence of the radiogenic cell death of endocrine tissue.

Thus ionizing radiation poses a threat to humans because it can cause a wide range of serious somatic illnesses. The experience of threat, in turn, is central to the production of psychological stress in human beings. The predominant theoretical model in the field of stress, which is known as the stress and coping paradigm, tells us that psychological stress occurs only when people encounter events that they regard as threatening.[6] Richard Lazarus expresses the centrality of threat to this analysis of stress when he says that "psychological stress analysis . . . is distinguished from other types of stress analysis by the intervening variable of threat."[7]

Within the stress and coping model, the word threat has a specific technical meaning. A preliminary definition of threat is that it is a psychological state in which a person has decided, by virtue of a variety of cognitive operations, that a present event indicates that something harmful will be happening in the future. In Lazarus's words, "Its main characteristics are two-fold: (1) it is anticipatory or future-oriented and (2) it is brought about by cognitive processes involving perception, learning memory judgment and thought."[8] In a more common sense fashion, an event is held to be threatening if the person experiencing that event judges it to be an indication that future events will be occurring that will be harmful to that person. In summary, "threat implies a state in which the individual anticipates a confrontation with a harmful condition of some sort."[9]

The stress and coping paradigm gives a thorough description of the psychological processes that a person uses to determine whether a given event is threatening. The paradigm also provides a formal description of the processes by which a person can come to master a threatening or potentially threatening situation. We will be using this paradigm to describe and analyze the psychosocial effects of invisible environmental contaminants.

In particular, we will use this model to take a careful look at the cognitive response of human beings to ambiguous threatening events of a chronic and enduring nature. This is of particular relevance to our inquiry because, as we have already seen, exposure to any of the invisible contaminants has the capacity to immerse a person in a threatening situation that persists and is enduringly ambiguous. Exposure to an invisible contaminant often generates threatening situations in which the meaning of the threatening event and its consequences can remain uncertain for long periods of time.

In looking at the psychological assessment of threatening events that are both ambiguous and enduring, our intent is to (1) gain an empirical and analytical understanding of the cognitive effects of the invisible contaminants and (2) look at the effect of chronic stimulus ambiguity on a person's ability to master the threat embodied in that ongoing situation.

The stress and coping paradigm appears to have emerged as the principal explanatory model of psychological stress. Psychological stress, as opposed to physiological stress, results from a psychological determination that a particular event, for example, being fired from one's job, is threatening. Physiological stress, as studied by Hans Selye, results from an organism's physiological determination that a particular event, for example, inoculation with a toxin, is threatening to the health of that organism.[10]

Lazarus's work on psychological stress began with the question: "Under what conditions of stress does deterioration of functioning occur?"[11] In other words, he was attempting to understand how stress causes the deterioration of cognitive and behavioral responses to threatening situations. In the process of investigating this question, Lazarus discovered that stress does not always lead to a deterioration in the quality of adaptation. Instead, he found "that three kinds of results occurred under stress: (1) no measureable effect (2) impairment of performance and (3) facilitation [of performance]."[12] These findings eventually led him to the formulation of a "cognitive-phenomenological" and interactive model of stress and coping. The resulting stress and coping paradigm can also be used to explain a larger class of phenomena: the emotions.[13]

The stress and coping paradigm is a thorough embodiment of the idea that psychological stress is the consequence of a more or less cognitive interaction between a person and either an environmental or psychological event.

Stress can not be defined exclusively by situations because the capacity of any situation to produce stress reactions depends on the characteristics of the individual. Similarly, stress reactions in an individual do not provide adequate grounds for defining the situation associated with it as a stress. . . . An observation of Janis is typical and relevant. He found that the intensity of preoperative fear in patients anticipating surgery was not correlated . . . with the objective seriousness of the operation. The important role of personality factors in producing stress reactions requires that we define stress in terms of *transactions* between individuals and situations, rather than of either one in isolation.[14]

It is worth pausing for a moment over this last passage. It has particular relevance to understanding the psychological effects of the invisible environmental contaminants. Lazarus's interactionist position stands in distinct contrast to what can be called the objectivist position regarding stress. The objectivist position holds that there is an objective, or appropriate, if you will, amount of stress in a given situation. The appropriate amount of stress is somehow a function of the objective characteristics of a stressful event. An objectivist might hold, for example, that it is appropriate to be threatened by some events, perhaps a diagnosis of cancer, but that it is not appropriate to be threatened by other events, perhaps a nuclear power plant accident.

Such distinctions and judgments are actually not objective in the usual sense of the word. Judgments of this type must be made relative to the objectivist's own sense of what is and is not threatening. The stress and coping paradigm avoids this objectivist fallacy by regarding stress and threat as the consequence of an interaction between a person and a potentially threatening event.

The description, then, of psychological stress within this paradigm begins with an enunciation of the three variables used to describe this interaction: an independent variable, an intervening variable and a dependent variable. It is important to be precise about the definition of stress because there has been historically considerable confusion about the meaning of the term.[15] In addition, there is some sense of conflict between the common sense and scientific meaning of the word stress.

Within the stress and coping paradigm, the word stress is "a generic term for the whole area of problems that includes the stimuli producing stress reactions, the reactions themselves and the various intervening processes."[16] In this formulation, the word stress seems to lose its common sense meaning. Instead of being something akin to an unpleasant effect of a difficult situation, stress becomes, instead, something entirely different: an area of study. However, if one takes a closer look at this "area of problems" definition, one finds that the definition simply spells out and teases apart the three variables that interact to produce the unpleasant effect that laymen understand to be stress.

I would like to briefly reconcile this "area of problems" definition with common sense notions of stress. The three variables to which the technical definition refers are (1) the stimuli producing stress reactions, or the stressor, (2) the stress reactions themselves, and (3) the various psychological responses intervening between the stressor and the responses to that stressor. The experience of stress is the result of an interaction between these three variables.

The three-variable analysis implies a sequence of events that produce the experience of stress. This sequence of events can be represented schematically as follows:

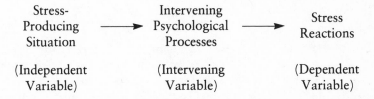

In light of the objectivist fallacy and the importance of conceiving of stress as an interaction between a stressful situation and a person, the diagram suggests that experimental stress is produced in the following manner:

1. A potentially threatening event occurs (independent variable).
2. The person experiencing the event decides, through the use of a number of cognitive processes, that the event is a threat to health and/or welfare (intervening variable).
3. The person has, as a consequence of this cognitive evaluation, a number of stress reactions to the event.

Within this paradigm, the experience of stress is simply one reaction that a person has to a situation that he or she judges to be threatening.

The paradigm suggests that stress is the experience of being threatened by a situation, that being threatened results in a number of psychological and physiological responses to that situation, that a number of cognitive processes are involved in the process of determining that a given situation is threatening, and that a person's determination that a particular situation is threatening is a function of two basic variables: (1) the nature of the event itself and (2) the personality of the individual experiencing that event.

The stimuli, or independent variables, that produce stress reactions are the threatening situations that cause a person to experience the unpleasant effect of stress. The stress literature tells us that many types of events can cause stress reactions. Some stressful events are: (1) flying military combat missions, (2) imminent surgery, (3) parachute jumping, (4) living in a concentration camp, (5) the death of a loved one, and (6) taking a doctoral dissertation examination. The common denominator in these situations that cause a stress reaction is that they are all situations in which people's most important values and goals [are] endangered or disrupted."[17]

The dependent variables in stress are called the stress reactions. These reactions, or responses, are the (physiological and psychological) changes that occur in people who see themselves as being threatened by a given event. These reactions are both indicators that a person is experiencing stress, and they also play a role in creating the experience of stress, itself. Four categories of stress response to perceived threat have been delineated:[18]

1. The experience of disturbed effects, including fear, anxiety, anger, depression, and guilt.

2. Physiological stress responses, including increased secretion of adreno-cortical hormones, and increased autonomic nervous system activity as evidenced in the altered activity of the end-organs controlled and modulated by the autonomic nervous system. End-organ responses that have been traditionally considered to be indicators of stress are galvanic skin response, blood pressure, heart rate, and respiratory rate.

3. Motor stress reactions, including increased muscle tension, speech disturbances, and certain facial expressions.

4. Changes in cognitive functioning, including either improvements or impairments in cognitive functioning.

Finally, the intervening variables in this stress production dynamic are the psychological processes by which a person determines whether or not an event is threatening and how to adapt to and cope with that event. In the stress and coping paradigm, this evaluative process is conceived of as including a number of ongoing and interactive cognitive processes. These cognitive processes are known as primary appraisal, secondary appraisal, and reappraisal. This formal analysis of the cognitive processes that mediate and create the experience of stress was introduced into the field of stress studies with the appearance of the stress and coping paradigm in the 1960s. Prior to the emergence of this paradigm, individual differences in stress responses were believed to be a consequence of a person's motivational and emotional traits.[19]

"From the outset, the guiding outlook [of the stress and coping paradigm] was that stress could not be defined at the stimulus level alone, but depended on the ways environmental events were construed by the individual, that is, their appraised significance for well being, and on the coping resources and options available and used."[20] Appraisal is not a single discrete event. It "consists of a continuously changing set of judgments about the significance of the flow of events for the person's well being. . . . Cognitive appraisal can be simply understood as the mental process of placing any event in one of a series of evaluative categories related either to its significance for the person's well being [primary appraisal] or to the available coping resources and options [secondary appraisal]."[21] In other words, the appraisal of environmental events involves a process of gathering and analyzing information about self and environment that enables a person to evaluate the significance of an event for his or her welfare.

This process of constructing an appraisal of environmental events and placing them in evaluative categories begins with the cognitive process of primary appraisal. Primary appraisal is defined as "the process of evaluating the significance of a transaction [with the environment] for one's well being."[22] Primary appraisal renders an event as belonging to one of three possible evaluative categories: (1) irrelevant, (2) benign-positive, or (3) harmful. For example, in primary appraisal one might decide that a forest fire located twenty miles away is of no immediate threat to one's house. A person living on a coastal island might decide that an approaching hurricane at a distance of one hundred miles poses sufficient threat to life and limb to warrant evacuation from that island.

The second basic form of event evaluation is called by Lazarus secondary appraisal.[23] "The word secondary does not mean that it necessarily follows primary appraisal in time or is less important."[24] In fact, "secondary appraisal and primary appraisal processes are interdependent, and even seem to fuse. Their only difference consists of the contents to which they are addressed."[25] Secondary appraisal refers to those cognitive processes in which a person considers and evaluates the range of coping responses available for adapting to a particular threatening situation. Primary appraisal, in contrast, involves an evaluation of the threatening event itself.

For example, the secondary appraisal of a sailing accident might involve an assessment of whether or not it is better to remain with a sinking boat or to attempt to swim through strong tidal currents to a distant shore. In a movie theatre fire it might involve an assessment of whether or not to leave by the side or back door, or whether it is necessary to stand up and attempt to calm down the panicking crowd.

Secondary appraisal, then, is the process by which a person decides how to adapt to an event to which an adaptation is deemed necessary. However, "secondary appraisal is [not only] important in shaping the coping activities of the person under psychological stress, [it also plays a role] in shaping the primary appraisal process itself."[26] It seems obvious that secondary appraisal affects primary appraisal if one considers a more recent definition of stress by Lazarus and Launier: "'Stress' is any event in which environmental or internal demands (or both) tax or exceed the adaptive resources of an individual, social system or tissue system."[27] Thus determination of whether or not an event is threatening depends at least in part on an assessment of whether or not adequate resources are available to master the situation.

The third cognitive process brought to bear upon the appraisal of potentially threatening events is known as reappraisal. Reappraisal is just that: it is an alteration of a prior primary or secondary appraisal as a consequence of either new information about a threatening event or feedback about the consequences of one's attempts at adaptation. For example, if a hurricane suddenly veers away from land and moves toward sea, the island dweller will then perceive its threat to him as substantially reduced. The sailor who left his small and sinking dinghy to swim for shore might reappraise his situation and return to his dinghy when he discovers that it is impossible to make progress toward shore because the current against which he is swimming is too strong.

The adaptational import of the appraisal and reappraisal processes lies in the fact that they mediate and inform a person's coping responses to a threatening situation. "Coping consists of efforts, both action oriented and intrapsychic, to manage (i.e., master, tolerate, reduce, minimize) environmental and internal demands, and conflicts among them, which tax or exceed a person's resources."[28] Coping with a threat might involve taking direct action (such as putting out a fire) or gathering information about the threat in question. If a coping strategy is successful, it will most likely reduce threat and stress reactions to that threat. If a coping strategy is unsuccessful, threat and stress reduction will not occur.

Coping behaviors have two major functions: (1) instrumental functions and (2) the regulation of emotions.[29] Coping behaviors that have an instrumental function alter or seek to alter a situation so that it is no longer threatening. Coping behaviors that regulate emotions attempt to reduce stress reactions to a threatening situation in order to (1) improve the likelihood of successful adaptation and (2) curtail the negative psychosomatic effects of those reactions.

There are also four modes, or categories, of coping behavior. The four modes are: (1) information seeking, (2) direct action, (3) inhibition of action, and (4) intrapsychic modes. The gathering of information has two basic functions. It can give a person the information necessary to adapt to a threatening situation, and the mere possession of information about a threat can also give a person a greater sense of mastery in regard to that threat—a sense that the situation is under control. Information can also be used to bolster previous threat-related decisions.[30] Hamburg and Adams have found that information-seeking behavior is part of the coping response to many different threat situations.[31].

It should also be noted that in some situations people will deliberately avoid the acquisition of new information about a threat. This is most often the case in situations involving injuries that are thought to be irreversible. In such circumstances, people will sometimes prefer to preserve the ambiguity present in a situation as a means of maintaining the hope and the will necessary to pursue additional attempts to adapt to the problem at hand.[32] "When little can be done to change the situation, the preservation of uncertainty can facilitate hope, morale, and involvement with living and help the person tolerate or relieve pain and emotional distress."[33] This strategy of the preservation of ambiguity has been seen, for example, in surgical patients.[34]

One finds, then, that in some stressful situations, a person will prefer to preserve ambiguity, but that in other threatening situations a person will prefer to gather as much information as possible about the nature of the threat.[35] The central determinant of whether a threatened person seeks ambiguity or information seems to lie in the nature of the threat. If a person believes that he or she cannot escape the injury foreshadowed by a threat, he or she will tend to seek ambiguity.[36] This idea is embodied in the stress response mode of defensive avoidance—one of the five types of behavioral response to threat delineated by Janis in his conflict model of decision making.[37]

On the other hand, if a person believes that escape from the injury prophesied by a threatening stimulus is possible, that person will seek the information requisite for successful appraisal of and adaptation to that threat. The pursuit of information in the face of avoidable threat can be seen in the two of the threat response categories delineated by Janis: vigilance and hypervigilance. Both of these responses, unlike defensive avoidance, are predicated on the belief that it is possible to find a better adaptation to the threat at hand.[38]

The collection of useful information in response to threatening situations involving exposures to an invisible environmental contaminant is often a difficult affair. Because of the invisibility of these contaminants, it is often impossible to gather the information necessary to make an empirically informed adaptation to that exposure. This has been the case, for example, in exposures involving a methyl alcohol contamination of illegally distilled whiskey,[39] an industrial carbon monoxide contamination,[40] military and commercial radiation-producing technology,[41] and a variety of contaminations involving toxic chemicals.[42] As we have already seen, the medical and environmental invisibility of certain contaminants makes it virtually impossible for anyone to gather the information needed either to appraise or to adapt to an invisible exposure. This lack of information produces, in turn, characteristic cognitive responses to these exposures. We will return to an investigation of these responses in later chapters.

In addition to providing an analysis of the phenomenon of stress and coping, the stress and coping paradigm also provides a model of the psychological processes by which the successful mastery of a threatening situation is accomplished. The process of mastery, as delineated by this paradigm, is a process that involves an appraisal of and an adaptation to a threatening event. The process of mastery has the same basic structure as the process that generates both the experience of stress and stress reactions. It involves the primary appraisal of threat, the secondary appraisal of coping options, and ongoing and constant reappraisal of threat and coping options in light of feedback from both the consequences of previous coping behavior and the changes that are occurring in the threatening situation.

For an example, imagine that you are restacking a pile of milled redwood slabs at your cabin in the mountains. As you pick up the last three slabs, a Pacific Coast Rattlesnake leaps out from underneath the slabs. You drop those slabs in absolute fear and leap backward away from the snake. You are scared and you are not certain what to do because you have never dealt with a rattlesnake before. Your heart is pounding as the rattlesnake crawls back under the abandoned redwood slabs. You stop, with this pause in the action, to assess the situation.

At this point, you have partaken in both primary and secondary appraisal. You decided that the snake is threatening (primary appraisal) and you also decided to depart from the situation (secondary appraisal) by putting some distance between you and the snake.

You consider forgetting the rattlesnake and going on with your business. After all, you can no longer see him. However, you quickly dismiss that option because you are going to be living at your cabin for the larger portion of the summer and the chances seem very good that either you or your loved ones will be making the acquaintance of the snake again. It is better, you decide, to do something about it now.

You begin to look around for weapons with which to attack the snake. You settle upon a shovel because it is long enough to keep an adequate distance between you and the snake. You decide to try and cut the snake in half with the edge of the shovel. In the back of your mind, you realize that you can always run if need be. You remind yourself not to let the snake get too close. All of these considerations are elaborate secondary appraisal.

Finally, you walk over to the slabs with your shovel and fling them aside. The snake draws up into a coil as if preparing to attack. You go through with your plans and begin to flail away at the snake with your weapon. Your heart is beating fast, and once again you are very scared (primary appraisal). Your repeated attempts to strike the snake miss the mark and he runs for cover under a second pile of wood.

You briefly realize that you missed the snake with the shovel because you were too scared to take careful aim (reappraisal), but the adrenalin is running very thick in your blood and you find yourself careening over toward the second pile of wood. You fling the wood aside with two gargantuan efforts and commence to beating the snake again. This time you find the mark and manage to cut the snake into pieces. Eventually you bury the snake, and peace slowly returns to your heart as you realize that you have achieved a mastery over the threat posed by the snake. After a brief rest, you return to the task of stacking the redwood slabs.

Adapting to and mastering the threat posed by the rattlesnake clearly involved the type of cognitive appraisal processes described by the stress and coping paradigm. One of the central contentions of the stress and coping paradigm is that the cognitive appraisal of threatening situations plays a necessary and indispensable role in the process of coping with those threatening situations.[43] As Shalit has said, "Adequate perceptual process is a prerequisite for adequate coping."[44]

Coping with and mastering a threatening event can, and often does, require a considerable amount of information. In the words of Folkman, Schaeffer, and Lazarus, "Certain information is needed to appraise accurately the significance of any transaction for one's well-being: The imminence of the transaction, the goals or commitments that are at risk, the probable outcome(s) or consequences, and what can be done to control the outcome."[45] Among other assessments, the protagonist in the rattlesnake narrative had to determine if the snake actually was a rattlesnake, whether or not he wanted to kill it, and whether or not he had the means at hand to kill the snake without getting bitten, and perhaps killed himself. The fact that adaptation to a threat is mediated by a cognitive process has been demonstrated in a laboratory setting. We need not rely solely on common sense or field observation to prove to ourselves that this is the case. The most convincing work in this regard is a series of laboratory studies done by Lazarus and his colleagues of film-induced stress.[46]

The question remains, however, as to what happens to the appraisal and coping process when the threatening events in question are of an ambiguous nature, and furthermore, what happens to these processes when this ambiguity and its resultant uncertainty persist for long periods of time? In considering the nature of the psychological effects of the invisible environmental contaminants, these are the questions that will have to be addressed and answered. The effects of chronically ambiguous and yet significant threat on the appraisal and coping processes will teach us much about the psychological effects of the invisible contaminants because, as we have already seen, exposure to these contaminants can immerse a person in an endless quandary of uncertainties about the meaning of that exposure.

Adaptation to a certain and palpable threat presents a person or persons with a considerably different set of problems than does adaptation to an uncertain or impalpable threat. If two people are standing in the street talking with one another, and both of them look up to find a truck barrelling down on them out of control, a clear course of successful adaptive behavior will probably become apparent to the two conversants. However, if the same two people were standing in the same street and they were told by a public health official that radiation had just been released into their environs by a nearby nuclear power plant accident, they may or may not know what they should do to protect themselves. They might decide to finish their conversation, or to go indoors to reduce exposure, or to evacuate the area with all due haste.

In coming to an understanding of the psychological effects of invisible contaminants, one of the central questions then becomes: given that the cognitive appraisal of the threat and the coping options is an indispensable element of coping with a threatening event, what happens to the appraisal process when the empirical information needed for such an appraisal is not available?

The answer, put briefly, is that for the most part the appraisal process proceeds just as though the necessary empirical information were actually available. Recall, for a moment, the cognitive response of medieval Europeans to the Plague, or the Chinese response to cholera, or the nineteenth-century European response to tuberculosis. All of these situations are good examples of how the appraisal of invisible threats, in this case medical threats, proceeds even though the empirical information germane to such an appraisal process is not available. In each of these situations, nonempirical belief systems were either invoked or created to explain the etiology of an illness caused by an invisible environmental contaminant. The same response also occurs in contemporary exposures to the invisible contaminants.

11
Nonempirical Belief Systems

F rom a modern viewpoint, it seems more than believable that fourteenth-century Europeans might go to great mythological lengths to explain the etiology of the Plague. Nor is it difficult for us to imagine that the South African Zulus would do much the same thing regarding the causes of tuberculosis. It is sobering, however, to remember that much of the educated opinion in nineteenth-century Europe, despite the positivism of the Enlightenment, believed that tuberculosis was a disease that descended on and was the result of a certain kind of rebellious, lamenting, and romantic personality.[1]

Each of these historic examples of the appraisal of the etiology of an invisible disease can be understood, in retrospect, as a nonempirical assessment of the medical threats posed by an invisible environmental contaminant. They were nonempirical because they were not based on actual observations of the causal agents of these diseases (*Pasteurella pestis* and *Mycobacterium tuberculosis*), nor were they grounded in the empirical study of other aspects of the resultant illness.

We cannot, however, dismiss these examples of the nonempirical appraisal of medical threats as a mere relic of past centuries and prescientific societies. It is tempting to assume that this is the case. After all, it can only seem incredible to us that persons from our own scientific age, persons familiar with the scientific method and the various fruits of its constant companion technology, would resort to the nonempirical assessment of a serious threat to their health and/or welfare. It seems only obvious that people would do far better to derive such an appraisal from careful observation of the threatening events in question. After all, if you are faced with a serious threat to your welfare, would you not want to predicate your response to that threat on the best available information?

Of course, it turns out to that the construction of nonempirical appraisals of medical threats is a frequent occurrence among peoples living in modern and scientific societies. As we will see, the nonempirical assessment of threats occurs in both scientific and pre-scientific societies. Given that this is the case, it becomes difficult to conclude, then, that nonempirical appraisals of threat are a consequence of ignorance, irrationality, and the like. They do not seem to occur as a result of a lack of familiarity with science. They appear, instead, to be an integral part of the process of coping with and adapting to invisible threats. The construction of nonempirical assessments of invisible threats appears to be a regularly occurring part of the appraisal of threats for which adequate information is not available. These assessments actually comprise and become the content of the cognitive appraisals that make adaptation to such threats possible. At times, they may even be based on rudimentary scientific observation.

Content of Nonempirical Belief Systems

Five studies have documented the development of nonempirical belief systems in contemporary populations that have been exposed to the invisible environmental contaminants. Four of these studies have actually described the thematic contents of these nonempirical belief systems, and one of them has strongly suggested the presence of such a belief system without describing its contents.[2] In addition, several studies of the psychological effects of the Three Mile Island accident have documented the prevalence of nonempirical appraisals of the health effects of that accident in members of the exposed population.[3]

The contents of these nonempirical belief systems concern the nature and consequences of the invisible exposures to which they are a cognitive response. As such, they comprise appraisals of the threat posed by the invisible contaminants to which the individuals in these populations have been exposed. The four invisible exposures for which nonempirical appraisals have been documented are as follows:

1. The exposure of the Love Canal population to the several toxic chemicals buried in the Love Canal.[4]
2. The exposure of military personnel to ionizing radiation as a consequence of their participation in atmospheric nuclear weapons tests.[5]
3. The occupational exposure of industrial workers to toxic chemicals.[6]
4. The exposure of the Three Mile Island area population to ionizing radiation as the result of a nuclear power plant accident.[7]

Each of the belief systems constructed around these exposures is nonempirical because it contains appraisals of an invisible threat based on conclusions for which empirical data were simply not available.

Belief systems constructed in response to an exposure to an invisible environmental contaminant portray a consistent picture of the exposure and its consequences. They describe the exposure as having been either safe or dangerous. They almost always describe the medical consequences of that exposure, but often, as we shall see, they are concerned with a much larger spectrum of issues.

Consider, for example, the belief system developed by some of the military veterans exposed to ionizing radiation while participating in atmospheric nuclear weapons tests. This belief system is concerned with a number of matters related to their radiation exposure, and it was developed as part of their process of coping with the illnesses they were developing fifteen to thirty years after their exposure. They developed their belief systems independently of one another and began to do so only after they developed somatic illnesses they thought might be related to their exposure to radiation.

The major thematic consistencies found in the atomic veteran belief system have been described as follows:[8]

1. A belief that they are dying of a disease caused by radiation

2. A belief that they will die early

3. A disrespect for the medical profession as a whole because it has been unable and sometimes unwilling to help

4. A longing to find that one doctor who will have all the answers

5. A heightened concern for the future health of their children and grand-children

6. Anger at the government, based on the belief that the government knowingly placed them in a dangerous situation and is now refusing to accept responsibility

7. Guilt over their anger at the government

8. The belief that they were used as guinea pigs

9. A willingness to be in the service again

10. A refusal to ever be involved with nuclear weapons again

11. The belief that most people think they are crazy for believing that ionizing radiation is dangerous and/or the cause of their illness.

The atomic veteran belief system portrays an invisible exposure as having been dangerous, but there can also be considerable variation in the contents of the belief systems developed in response to a single invisible exposure. Some people construct a belief system that portrays the exposure as an exceedingly dangerous event.[9] Others construct a belief system that portrays the exposure as a nonevent that will have little or no negative effect upon their health and welfare.[10] It seems to be the case that exposure to an invisible environmental contaminant will not, of necessity, generate belief systems that portray an invisible exposure as being either dangerous or safe. In fact, it appears that both types of belief systems are likely to appear in a population exposed to an invisible contaminant.[11]

Consider, for example, Fowlkes and Miller's work on the belief systems that developed in the Love Canal area population. Basically, they found that two polarized and mutually exclusive belief systems regarding the health effects of the canal were present in the population that lived in the area. One of these belief systems was held by a group of area residents that the authors call "believers."[12] This belief system portrayed the Love Canal dump site as a serious threat to the health of area residents. The component themes of this belief system are as follows:

1. The migration of the chemicals into the Love Canal neighborhood from the dump site was widespread.
2. The health effects of those chemicals are likely to be serious.
3. There has been an excessive number of cancers in the Love Canal neighborhood.
4. Those cancers have been caused by chemicals from the dump site.
5. There has been an excessive amount of noncancerous illness present in the Love Canal neighborhood.
6. This noncancerous illness has also been caused by the chemicals from the dump site.
7. My family's health problems have been caused by the chemicals from the dump site.
8. The doctors don't understand our health problems.
9. Government officials generally tried to minimize the problem.
10. Those politicians who helped the Love Canal area residents did so in order to get votes.

The second belief system was held by a group of area residents that the authors called "nonbelievers."[13] This belief system portrayed the dump site as posing a minimal threat to the health of area residents. The component themes of this belief system are as follows:

1. The migration of chemicals into the Love Canal neighborhood from the dump site has been minimal.
2. The health effects of the chemicals located in the dump site are also minimal.
3. The health problems of people in this neighborhood were not caused by the chemicals in the Love Canal.

4. These health problems can and do happen everywhere. They are not unique to this neighborhood.

5. The people who are worried about Love Canal are too emotional.

6. The people who are concerned about Love Canal are radicals and opportunists.

In a study of community reaction to the Love Canal disaster, Levine found a third type of belief system present in the Love Canal area population. She found that the believer group had developed a belief system concerning the nature of the predicament. The thematic consistencies of that belief system are as follows:[14]

1. We are victims of a disaster.

2. The problems we face are too large for us. We need help.

3. We are good citizens. We deserve help from the government.

4. The government can and should help us now.

5. We are being treated unfairly.

6. We must stick together to take care of ourselves.

7. Family and community help is not enough for our needs.

8. No one but the government has enough resources for our pressing needs.

9. We must work together to force the government to provide what we are entitled to.

Studies of the psychological effects of the Three Mile Island accident also provide evidence of the role that nonempirical beliefs play in the appraisal of invisible threats. These studies also demonstrate the abundant variation that occurs in the appraisal of an invisible exposure. As we shall be seeing, some of the Three Mile Island area residents adamantly believe that the radiation released from Three Mile Island poses no threat to their health and welfare. Other area residents believe with equal tenacity that the accident has already had and will continue to have serious negative effects on their health.[15]

Consider, for example, the results of a survey by Houts et al. of the TMI area population.[16] The survey was done in October 1980, nineteen months after the accident. Houts's researchers included six statements that they called rumors in a larger survey and asked two groups of subjects whether they agreed or disagreed with these rumors. One group of subjects was composed of people living within five miles of TMI. The second group was composed of people living between forty-one and fifty-five miles from the plant. The results show that: (1) the vast majority of the subjects had already reached conclusions about the health effects of the accident, and (2) there was considerable variation in the conclusions to which people had come. Frequency

Table 11–1
Rumors from the Houts's Study of TMI Area Residents
(percent of responses)

	0–5 Miles from TMI	41–55 Miles from TMI
There has been an increase in the number of miscarriages, stillborns, and infant deaths since the TMI accident.		
Definitely	9	13
Probably	26	34
Don't know	10	11
Probably not	40	32
Definitely not	15	10
There has been an increase in birth defects in the area since TMI.		
Definitely	7	12
Probably	24	33
Don't know	13	8
Probably not	41	38
Definitely not	15	9
Cancer rates will increase in the area because of TMI.		
Definitely	17	11
Probably	37	45
Don't know	7	9
Probably not	32	27
Definitely not	7	8
Farm animals in the area have had an increase in health problems since TMI.		
Definitely	16	14
Probably	32	45
Don't know	7	9
Probably not	34	23
Definitely not	11	9

Source: Peter Houts et al., "Health Related Behavioral Impact of the Three Mile Island Nuclear Incident," Part I (Submitted to the Three Mile Island Advisory Panel of Health Research Studies of the Pennsylvania Department of Health, 1981).

distributions of the responses to four of these rumors are presented in table 11–1.

In 1980 and 1981 the Field Research Corporation was commissioned to do several public opinion polls of the TMI area population.[17] A June 1980 poll contained two questions regarding the perceived health effects of the accident. Again, two study groups were polled: one living within five miles of the plant and one living between five and twenty-five miles from the plant. The questions and their responses are presented in table 11–2.

Table 11–2
Field Research Corporation Questions of TMI Area Residents
(percent of responses)

	0–5 Miles from TMI	5–25 Miles from TMI
Do you believe that you got a dangerous dose of radiation during the TMI accident?		
Yes	14	8
No	60	72
Don't know	25	19
Not in area	1	1
Do you stand a chance of getting a dangerous dose of radiation from TMI sometime in the future?		
Yes	49	41
No	32	39
Don't know	19	20

Source: Field Research Corporation, Public Opinion in Pennsylvania toward the Accident at Three Mile Island and Its Aftermath (San Francisco: Field Research Corporation, 1980).

In August 1982 I surveyed a study group composed of TMI area residents living within five miles of the plant and of a control group of individuals living within the same distance of the Calvert Cliffs nuclear power plant in Calvert Cliffs, Maryland. The Calvert Cliffs sample was chosen as a control group because the Calvert Cliffs plant has no history of a major or visible accident. Some of the results of this study are presented in the tables below. Basically, the study found that TMI area residents had already accomplished considerable appraisal of the threats posed by the TMI accident.[18] For example, as shown in table 11–3, area residents had reached conclusions about the health effects of the accident in terms of increased miscarriages, childrens' illnesses, and potential cancers.

Residents had also developed beliefs about the environmental effects of the accident. As shown in table 11–4, they had reached conclusions about the effects of the accident on the air, earth, plants, and flowers.

TMI area residents were also asked about doses of radiation they received from TMI. The results are shown in table 11–5.

Finally, TMI residents reported having a decreased sense of security and safety about living in the area and a decreased sense of trust in governmental authorities as a result of the accident. Table 11–6 presents the responses made to questions that touched upon these issues.

The results of this survey also suggest that two different subpopulations within the TMI area population have developed two entirely different but coherent belief systems about the consequences of the TMI accident. One subpopulation has constructed a belief system that portrays the accident as having had not deleterious effects upon the health of the TMI area popula-

Table 11–3
Beliefs about the Health Effects of the TMI Accident
(percent of responses)

	TMI	Calvert Cliffs
Women are having more miscarriages.		
Strongly agree	10.96	4.49
Somewhat agree	28.22	8.99
Somewhat disagree	32.60	32.58
Strongly disagree	28.22	53.93
Children are developing more illnesses.		
Strongly agree	19.47	9.38
Somewhat agree	27.36	9.38
Somewhat disagree	26.58	26.04
Strongly disagree	26.58	55.21
Farm animals are having more health problems.		
Strongly agree	23.45	6.32
Somewhat agree	27.22	16.84
Somewhat disagree	23.18	23.16
Strongly disagree	25.88	53.68
People are more likely to get cancer.		
Strongly agree	30.61	12.25
Somewhat agree	27.30	14.29
Somewhat disagree	19.89	23.47
Strongly disagree	22.19	50.00
I feel certain that it is only a matter of time until I or someone I know develops a cancer caused by radiation released from TMI.		
Strongly agree	23.90	9.38
Somewhat agree	18.70	9.38
Somewhat disagree	21.03	26.04
Strongly disagree	36.36	55.00
The amount of illness caused by radiation will increase if TMI reopens.		
Strongly agree	25.13	3.09
Somewhat agree	20.42	15.46
Somewhat disagree	16.75	26.80
Strongly disagree	37.70	54.64

Source: H.M. Vyner, "The Psychosocial Effects of the Invisible Environmental Contaminants" (Presented at the Three Mile Island Public Health Fund's Workshop on the Psychosocial Effects of the Invisible Environmental Contaminants, June 1984).
Note: $p = .0001$

tion. A second subpopulation appears to have constructed a belief system that portrays the accident as both having and continuing to have serious untoward effects upon the health and welfare of the TMI area population. A third subpopulation seems to have reached inconsistent conclusions about the effects of the accident.[19]

Table 11–4
Beliefs about the Environmental Impacts of the TMI Accident
(percent of responses)

	TMI	Calvert Cliffs
The air and earth are contaminated, and are still giving off radiation.		
Strongly agree	21.39	4.09
Somewhat agree	31.19	8.99
Somewhat disagree	21.65	32.58
Strongly disagree	25.77	53.93
Plants and flowers do not grow normally.		
Strongly agree	15.24	4.04
Somewhat agree	14.99	7.07
Somewhat disagree	25.58	25.25
Strongly disagree	44.19	63.63

Source: H.M. Vyner, "The Psychosocial Effects of the Invisible Environmental Contaminants" (Presented at the Three Mile Island Public Health Fund's Workshop on the Psychosocial Effects of the Invisible Environmental Contaminants, June 1984).
Note: p = .0001

Table 11–5
Beliefs about the Doses of Radiation Released from the TMI Accident
(percent of responses)

	TMI
People living in the TMI area at the time of the accident were exposed to radiation.	
Strongly agree	40.66
Somewhat agree	34.60
Somewhat disagree	14.90
Strongly disagree	9.85
Radiation is still being released from TMI.	
Strongly agree	33.25
Somewhat agree	35.30
Somewhat disagree	15.86
Strongly disagree	15.60
If Unit One (TMI) reopens, people living in the TMI area will be exposed to more radiation.	
Strongly agree	35.37
Somewhat agree	24.43
Somewhat disagree	16.03
Strongly disagree	24.17

Source: H.M. Vyner, "The Psychosocial Effects of the Invisible Environmental Contaminants" (Presented at the Three Mile Island Public Health Fund's Workshop on the Psychosocial Effects of the Invisible Environmental Contaminants, June 1984).

Table 11–6
Beliefs about Safety and Trust in Government after the TMI Accident
(percent of responses)

	TMI	Calvert Cliffs
I don't really feel safe here anymore.[a]		
Strongly agree	17.34	6.00
Somewhat agree	20.30	4.00
Somewhat disagree	15.54	15.00
Strongly disagree	46.62	75.00
I take precautions to protect myself from TMI.[b]		
Strongly agree	11.45	7.07
Somewhat agree	19.85	11.11
Somewhat disagree	23.92	12.12
Strongly disagree	44.78	69.70
I am angry at the Nuclear Regulatory Commission because they say that TMI is less dangerous than it is.[c]		
Strongly agree	32.15	16.33
Somewhat agree	19.75	23.47
Somewhat disagree	24.05	18.37
Strongly disagree	24.05	41.83
I have greater faith in the government and authorities in general.[d]		
Strongly agree	13.20	26.53
Somewhat agree	20.56	18.36
Somewhat disagree	27.66	26.53
Strongly disagree	35.58	28.57
I feel as though the accident is still going on.		
Strongly agree	22.65	
Somewhat agree	24.43	
Somewhat disagree	15.01	
Strongly disagree	37.91	

Source: H.M. Vyner, "The Psychosocial Effects of the Invisible Environmental Contaminants" (Presented at the Three Mile Island Public Health Fund's Workshop on the Psychosocial Effects of the Invisible Environmental Contaminants, June 1984).
Note: [a]$p = .0001$
[b]$p = .0006$
[c]$p = .0009$
[d]$p = .0002$

There is one additional study that documents the appearance of belief systems in a population exposed to an invisible contaminant. Brodsky did psychiatric evaluations of seventy patients who "believed that they had been injured by inhaling non-infectious, airborne substances in the workplace" who had "filed for workers compensation benefits for the injury."[20] All of the workers, when subjected to "traditional physical and psychiatric examination showed no evidence of physical damage or physical functional impairment attributable to the alleged exposure in the workplace."

Essentially, Brodsky's work is a study of patients who had adopted the self-diagnostic belief[21] that they had been physically injured by a toxic exposure. Brodsky does not directly discuss whether or not he believes his subjects reached this conclusion as a means of facilitating their application for workers' compensation. However, his presentation of their typical "illness career" gives the distinct impression that the two decisions were unrelated.

To be more specific, Brodsky divided his subjects into two groups on the basis of the type of "illness career path" they had followed before deciding they had been injured by a previous exposure. The first group of subjects decided that they had been injured by an occupational exposure after being involved in a discernable event involving accidental exposure to excessive amounts of a particular chemical. Brodsky found that this group of subjects reached the conclusion that they had been injured by the previous exposure when they developed unremitting and undiagnosable somatic and/or psychological symptoms.

The second group of subjects developed a self-diagnostic belief that a previous toxic exposure had harmed them "after a gradual and vague onset of inexplicable symptoms." In these cases, there was no specific event that the patient could identify as a moment at which an accidental exposure to toxic chemicals had occurred. However, with the persistence of their symptoms, each of these patients came to believe that his or her illness had been caused by ongoing exposure to toxic chemicals.

Brodsky does not describe in detail the themes of the belief systems developed by these patients. However, he does discuss the fact that in both groups, the belief that they had been injured by a toxic exposure became a central organizing principle in the believing persons' lives. Important aspects of their lives—including employment practices, health care, and the avoidance of a broad spectrum of potential contaminants—were a consequence of their self-diagnostic belief.

It can be seen, then, that individuals exposed to an invisible environmental contaminant will construct and adopt nonempirical appraisals and belief systems about the nature of that exposure. Some people develop nonempirical beliefs that portray the exposure as benign. This response has been documented at both Love Canal[22] and Three Mile Island.[23] Other exposed persons appraise an invisible exposure as a serious health threat. This response has been documented among residents of the Love Canal area,[24] residents of the TMI area,[25] military veterans exposed to radiation,[26] and workers occupationally exposed to toxic chemicals.[27]

This variation in belief system content is the predictable consequence of the invisibility, and thus ambiguity, of the invisible environmental contaminants. In threatening situations involving unambiguous events, the events themselves place some constraints on the interpretations and meanings that people will give to the threatening situation. However, in situations involving ambiguous threat, the events that comprise the situation place considerably less constraint on the meanings that different individuals will give to those stimuli. As a result, "ambiguity permits maximum latitude for idiosyncratic interpretations of situations."[28]

When situational constraints on the interpretation of events are not present, individual psychological factors play a greater role in determining the meanings given to those events. "Since the stimulus configuration cannot determine the appraisal because its significance is not clear, factors within the psychological structure have greater prominence in the appraisal."[29] Both Withey and Lazarus suggest that ambiguous stimuli will be interpreted in terms of a person's existing cognitive structure.[30] Withey emphasizes the determining influence of conditions at the time of the threatening event. Lazarus places more emphasis on the general beliefs that a person holds about transactions with the environment. He cites Erikson's concept of basic trust as an example of such a belief.

The Function of Nonempirical Belief Systems

We have observed that ignorance of the ways of science is not a prior condition for the construction of nonempirical belief systems about an invisible exposure. Why then do people create such belief systems? Do nonempirical belief systems serve any function that would explain their appearance and persistence in response to an invisible exposure?

One of several answers to this question is that the construction of nonempirical belief systems in response to an invisible threat may serve to reduce the stress caused by the ambiguity of the exposure situation. Ambiguity and uncertainty in and of themselves can be stressful.[31] Ambiguity and/or uncertainty seem to produce stress in human beings because they either diminish or totally obviate a person's ability to control a threatening or nonthreatening situation. Exposure to any of the invisible environmental contaminants places a person in a situation that is, as we have already seen, laden with ambiguity and uncertainty.

Evidence for the fact that ambiguity is stressful in and of itself comes from a number of sources. Several laboratory studies have shown that: (1) ambiguity is stressful, and (2) people prefer unambiguous situations to ambiguous ones. For example, Ball and Vogler found that 64 percent (25 of 39) of their subjects, when placed in an experimental situation in which receipt of an electric shock was inevitable, preferred to administer the shock themselves.[32] Subjects reported that they preferred self-administered shock to experimenter-administered shock because of the resultant "predictability of the shock." They preferred certainty and sense of control. Averill in a review of the major experiments that have investigated self-administered versus other-administered noxious stimuli found that most people prefer to have control over a potentially noxious stimulus.[33]

Additional evidence for the stressful nature of ambiguity can be found in the disaster literature.[34] Janis has collected a number of instances in which ambiguity, in the context of disaster situations, results in increased fear, anxiety, and vigilance among the victims of a disaster. He found evidence of this dynamic in disasters involving occupational exposure of factory workers to carbon monoxide,[35] underground gas explosions beneath a New York community,[36] methyl alcohol contamination of illegally distilled whiskey in Atlanta,[37] and posthurricane flooding of another New York community.[38]

In all of these situations, Janis found confirmation of what he calls an ambiguity hypothesis. He states this hypothesis as follows: "Under conditions where a serious warning has aroused fear to a moderate or high level, the recipient's vigilance tendencies will tend to be increased by any subsequent communication or physical sign that he perceives as containing ambiguous information about his vulnerability."[39] For example, in December 1952, workers in a Chicago factory were continuously exposed during the course of a work day to the invisible environmental contaminant carbon monoxide. In Janis's words, "This [industrial disaster] involved an unknown and undetectable causal agent, the insidious presence of which could be inferred only from the ill effects it produced in its victims."[40]

When the exposure first began in the morning of December 8, employees developed the symptoms of carbon monoxide asphyxiation: headache, nausea, dizziness, and weakness. At first, it was thought that the symptomatic workers were suffering from more common problems, such as the flu or hangovers. As the number of asphyxiation cases mounted, factory employees began to realize that something else was wrong, but that they could not see what it was. A frenzied search for the source of the invisible problem was initiated. As one factory employee said, "I got almost hysterical because I couldn't put my finger on what it was."[41]

Powell has described a similar hypervigilant response in the black community in Atlanta in response to invisible methyl alcohol contamination of a shipment to that community of illegally distilled whiskey. Janis regards this incident as additional evidence of the stress producing and enhancing effects of ambiguous information in threatening situations. He bases his assertion on the results of Powell's examination of the medical records of the 433 patients who reported to Grady Hospital seeking treatment for methyl alcohol poisoning. He found that 42 percent of these patients (n = 183) were completely asymptomatic; an additional 18 percent (n = 75) reported somatic symptoms for which no clinical verification could be obtained; and only 40 percent were actually found to be suffering from methyl alcohol poisoning. Janis regards these statistics as evidence that, among other reactions, ambiguous threats can cause hypervigilance and apprehension.[42]

A third type of evidence indicating that ambiguity is threatening and stress producing comes from a small group of clinical studies. Dibner found that psychiatric patients in an ambiguous clinical interview situation experienced more anxiety than patients in an unambiguous clinical interview situation.[43] Subjects in the unambiguous situation were constantly asked questions by their interviewer. Subjects in the ambiguous situation were simply told to talk about themselves. Dibner measured patient anxiety through the use of palmar skin conductance measures, anxiety cards, anxiety ratings from judges, and the clinical signs of anxiety in subject speech.

I found an intolerance of uncertainty among military veterans exposed to radiation.[44] The uncertainty surrounding the health effects of their exposures was a source of considerable discomfort for these men. As one veteran put it, "To get a bad diagnosis is better than receiving no diagnosis at all. Otherwise you keep wondering about it."[45] This expressed intolerance of uncertainty is reminiscent of Hudson's finding that in uncertain disaster situations some individuals say that "the worst would be better than this [uncertainty]."[46]

One last line of clinical evidence regarding the stress-producing properties of ambiguity comes from a study of the intolerance of ambiguity by Frenkel-Brunswick.[47] Frenkel-Brunswick found that some people are more intolerant of ambiguity than others. In her own words, "for many, mere exposure to a stimulus whose meaning is unclear is a source of threat." She concluded that this propensity to regard ambiguity as a threat is a personality trait.

It appears, then, that ambiguity constitutes a threat and also acts as an amplifier of existing threat because it renders control of a situation impossible. Situational ambiguity makes control difficult because it reduces a person's ability to appraise a threatening situation. As Shalit has stated, "It has been shown that failure to cope, in a variety of physical, social or psychological situations, is associated with increased ambiguity of the structure of those situations. . . . As ambiguity increases, coping potential decreases."[48] Lazarus takes the same position when he says that "ambiguity concerning the significance of a stimulus configuration will usually intensify threat because it limits the individual's sense of control or increases his sense of helplessness over the danger. But this occurs only when there are other grounds, either situational or characterological, for being threatened."[49] Finally, it has been demonstrated in a number of studies that the belief that one has lost control of a threatening situation can produce stress.[50]

Perhaps the most dramatic evidence of the stressful nature of not having control of a threatening situation is Seligman's work on learned helplessness.[51] Seligman has studied the response of human beings, as well as other species, to threatening situations from which escape is impossible. In these situations subjects learned that the outcome of their predicament was totally independent of their response to that situation.

Seligman calls the resultant pattern of behavior learned helplessness. The two primary symptoms of learned helplessness are: (1) passivity: "Subjects are slower to initiate responses to alleviate trauma and may not respond at all," and (2) retardation in learning, in situations in which escape is possible, that they can control the trauma being inflicted upon them. To illustrate the phenomenon of learned helplessness, Seligman presents us with the image of a dog lying motionless on the floor of a laboratory box and whining while receiving an electric shock from which it cannot escape.

Additional evidence of the stressful effects of the loss of control of a threatening situation comes from a study done by Geer, Davison, and Getchel.[52] They found that subjects who believed that they were in control of a threatening situation, even though they actually were not, had reduced anxiety in comparison to a group that did not think they were in control of the same situation.

To say that situational ambiguity causes both stress and loss of control is the same as saying that it is impossible to cope with a threatening situation unless it is possible to make a cognitive appraisal of that situation. Successful adaptation to a threatening situation requires the cognitive appraisal of that situation. There seems to be universal agreement on this point among students of stress. Consider, for example, Weiner's statement that "survival is guaranteed by the exquisite specificity and appropriateness of the response to a particular threat. In fact, when the threat is poorly defined—when an experience is ambiguous—an appropriate response can not be given. Fear is engendered because survival can not be assured in the absence of a behavioral program designed to overcome the threat."[53] Coping requires competent appraisal. Shalit makes this same point in saying that "effectiveness of coping in any situation will be related negatively to the structural ambiguity of that situation."[54]

Within this analysis of the relationship between cognitive appraisal, ambiguity, and the process of coping with threats, one finds the fundamental motive for the construction of nonempirical belief systems in response to an exposure to an invisible environmental contaminant. Competent adaptation to any threat requires the cognitive appraisal of that threat. Adaptation to a threatening situation is actually based upon the results of that appraisal. If a person is going to cope successfully with a threatening situation, that person must have reliable empirical information about the threat itself, the spectrum of available coping behaviors, and the available resources with which the threat can be mastered. If the information necessary for appraisal and coping is not available, a person can either (1) forego adaptation to that threat, or (2) construct an appraisal of the situation based upon whatever material is at hand and proceed to cope. In situations involving exposure to an invisible environmental contaminant, the information necessary for an appraisal is often not available because of the medical and environmental invisibility of the contaminant. Thus the construction of nonempirical belief systems arises as a means of appraising an exposure to an invisible contaminant. A belief system permits a person to adapt to the exposure.

A summary of this hypothesis has been put forth by Milburn and Watman in their book, *On the Nature of Threat*. In regard to the relationship between ambiguity, appraisal and coping, they wrote:

> In environments containing threats, organisms survive by reducing the randomness around them. Danger is implicit in unpredictability. . . . Organisms that reduce uncertainty have a survival advantage over those that do not reduce it effectively. This struggle against uncertainty can take many forms, but must fall into two general categories: efforts to reduce uncertainty by physical intervention in the environment, and efforts to reduce uncertainty by cognitively organizing and understanding the environment. . . . Both make life more predictable and, therefore, safer. . . . [Reducing uncertainty] can be understood as adjuncts to physical intervention. . . . Understanding a phenomenon . . . is a necessary precondition for physical control, [but] . . . reduction of uncertainty . . . is a powerful method, in its own right, of enlarging the human sphere of control beyond the range of physical instrumentalities.[55]

To be sure, the boundary between the activities of cognitive appraisal and coping can become a bit blurred. There are times when the process of appraisal actually becomes a means of coping with a threat. This transformation of appraisal behavior into coping behavior has been recognized in three types of cognitive activity. Lazarus has recognized the cognitive activity of defensive appraisal as a form of coping; Hamburg and Adams regard the seeking of information about a threat as a form of coping with that threat; and this book describes a third type of appraisal activity that becomes a form of coping: the construction of nonempirical belief systems in response to an exposure to an invisible environmental contaminant.

12
Hypervigilance

I rving L. Janis has elaborated a model that delineates and describes what he regards as the five basic behavioral and cognitive patterns of coping with stressful or threatening situations. His articulation of this model appears to have had its beginnings with his analysis of the psychological effects of disaster warnings[1] and to have subsequently matured into a more sophisticated model with his work on the stresses generated by decisional conflict. This later model is called the conflict theory model of decision making.[2]

Like Lazarus, the point of departure for Janis was the recognition that stress can, on the one hand, have decided adverse effects on the quality of adaptation to a threat, but that on the other hand "stress does not always have detrimental or maladaptive effects. On the contrary, anticipatory fear or excessive losses sometimes prevents premature closure. Such concerns can serve as incentives to carry out the adaptive 'work of worrying' which leads to careful information search and appraisal."[3]

In consequence of this recognition that stress can both promote and impede successful adaptations to threatening events, Janis has been interested in determining how to promote successful adaptations to stressful or threatening situations. In a 1962 paper entitled "Psychological Effects of Warnings," Janis states, "I have attempted to systematize what is now known about the conditions under which warnings and other preparatory communications are most effective in inducing adaptive behavior."[4] In *Decision Making,* Janis and Mann introduce their conflict theory model by saying, "Our theory attempts to specify the contrasting conditions that determine whether the stress engendered by decisional conflict will facilitate or interfere with vigilant information processing."[5] Vigilance, one of the five patterns of coping described by the Janis and Mann model, is regarded within that model as the most consistently adaptive mode of coping with threatening events. The vigilant decision maker will:

1. Thoroughly canvass a wide range of alternative courses of action;

2. Survey the full range of objectives to be fulfilled and the values implicated by the choice;

3. Carefully weigh whatever he knows about the costs and risks of negative consequences, as well as the positive consequences, that could flow from alternatives;

4. Intensively search for new information relevant to further evaluation of the alternatives;

5. Correctly assimilate and take account of any new information or expert judgment, even when the information or judgment does not support the course of action he or she initially prefers;

6. Reexamine the positive and negative consequences of all known alternatives before making a final choice;

7. Make detailed provisions for implementing or executing the chosen course of action, with special attention to contingency plans that might be required if various known risks were to materialize.

Janis and Mann extracted these criteria for vigilance from the literature on effective decision making.[6]

The remaining patterns of coping with threat, as portrayed within the conflict theory of decision making, are: (1) unconflicted inertia, (2) unconflicted change, (3) defensive avoidance, and (4) hypervigilance. These four additional modes of coping are seen as being "occasionally adaptive . . . especially for routine or minor decisions . . . but they often result in defective decision making when the decision maker is confronted with a vital choice that has serious consequences."[7]

Each of these coping patterns is characterized by a distinctive cognitive and behavioral response to threat. Janis characterizes them in the following manner:[8]

1. *Unconflicted Inertia.* The decision maker complacently decides to continue whatever he or she has been doing, ignoring information about associated risks.

2. *Unconflicted Change.* The decision maker uncritically adopts whichever new course of action is most salient or strongly recommended, without making contingency plans and without psychologically preparing for setbacks.

3. *Defensive avoidance.* The decision maker evades the conflict by procrastinating, by shifting responsibility to someone else, or by constructing wishful rationalizations that bolster the least objectionable alternative, minimizing the expected unfavorable consequences, and remaining selectively inattentive to corrective information.

4. *Hypervigilance.* The decision maker, in a panicky state, searches frantically for a way out of the dilemma, rapidly shifts back and forth between alternatives, and impulsively seizes upon a hastily contrived solution that seems to promise immediate relief. He or she overlooks the full range of consequences of his or her choice because of emotional excitement, repetitive thinking, and cognitive constriction.

Characteristics of Hypervigilance

In the analysis of the psychosocial effects of the invisible environmental contaminants, the pattern of coping with which we are most concerned, in addition to vigilance, is the pattern of hypervigilance. Hypervigilance is, in general, a consistent form of response to ambiguous threatening situations, and, in particular, a consistent form of response to exposures to the invisible environmental contaminants.

Hypervigilance comes in many forms. Janis regards panic as its most extreme form. For example, it is hypervigilance when people in a crowded and burning movie theater rush to the same exit simply because most everyone else is running to that exit, in ignorance of several other exits through which safe escape is possible. The hypervigilant response does not always reach such dramatic proportions. Janis regards the behavior of individuals reporting to an Atlanta emergency room for the treatment of methyl alcohol poisoning in the absence of genuine somatic symptoms as a form of hypervigilance.[9] As we will see, hypervigilance can also take the form of a preoccupation or obsession, if you will, with an ambiguous threat.

Janis and Mann conceive of hypervigilance as being the response "typically evoked in disasters when people fear imminent entrapment [as in a burning theater] because they see that they have very little time left in which to find a safe way out."[10] Lack of sufficient *time* to make adequate deliberations and choices is a central idea in Janis's formulation of the conditions that precipitate the hypervigilant response. The characteristics of hypervigilance are as follows:[11]

1. An excessive alertness to all signs of potential threat that results in a diffusion of attention;
2. A strong motivation to engage in a thorough search and appraisal;
3. Constant distraction from essential cognitive tasks by obsessional ideas about all the things that could go wrong;
4. Wasting of time and energy in maladaptive responses to the disaster because of indiscriminate attentiveness to all sorts of threats, both relevant and irrelevant;

5. A marked tendency toward stereotyped and oversimplified thinking about options;

6. The temporary loss of perceptual acuity, perceptual coordination, and motor skills.

In Janis's estimation, "the grossest errors in decisionmaking are to be expected whenever hypervigilance is the dominant stress reaction."[12]

Janis hypothesized that in addition to insufficient response time, ambiguous information about threat will also precipitate hypervigilance. He finds that in general, "under conditions where a serious warning has aroused fear to a moderate or high level, the recipient's vigilance tendencies will tend to be increased by any subsequent communication or physical sign that he perceives as containing ambiguous information about his vulnerability."[13] Thus, Janis himself has recognized that lack of time is not the only condition that will precipitate hypervigilance. That this is the case can be seen in several examples of hypervigilance that Janis presents.

Hypervigilance can occur as a response to ambiguous threats that do not involve exposure to an invisible environmental contaminant. For example, Janis regards the response of area residents to a disaster involving a series of underground gas explosions in Brighton, New York, as a form of hypervigilance.[14] In the week immediately following these explosions, area residents still did not understand the cause of those explosions and were prone to think that the worst was about to happen again. During that week, "many residents in and near the stricken neighborhood were jittery, unable to sleep, and constantly apprehensive about the possibility that the explosions might suddenly start again, despite repeated assurances from the authorities that the area was safe."[15]

As can be seen in this case, hypervigilance does not necessarily involve literal panic behavior. The behavior described as hypervigilance in this circumstance is an extreme form of vigilance behavior generated by a belief that more explosions were likely to happen. In this case, hypervigilance was a preoccupation with a potentially damaging event. The threatened individuals became preoccupied with danger because they knew that the invisibility of the threat made it almost impossible to cope with, or master, that threat should it actually recur. Since they did not know the cause of the previous explosions, they had no idea of whether more explosions would occur or how to prevent them. As a means of coping with this type of predicament, some individuals more or less assume that the unwanted and threatening event will occur. They take this approach as a means of optimizing vigilance and of maximizing the possibility of mastering the event. The result, as was the case at Brighton, is a hypervigilant preoccupation with the potentially harmful event.

Janis found another example of hypervigilant preoccupation with an ambiguous threat in the response of a group of Chicago factory workers to a carbon monoxide asphyxiation.[16] In this accident, the exposed workers initially responded to the invisible exposure by more or less ignoring it. At first they regarded the various symptoms reported by their fellow employees as the symptoms of routine illnesses of one sort or another. However, as more and more workers became seriously ill, hypervigilance set in. "The employees then became extremely agitated and stopped their business-as-usual activities to devote all their energies to discovering the source of the unknown danger and trying to escape from it."[17] In this particular event, we find, once again, that hypervigilance was manifest as an intense fear of and preoccupation with a threatening event.

The above examples are not isolated cases. Hypervigilance is a common response to exposures to an invisible environmental contaminant. Certainly this was the case with the Halbert family in Michigan, when their dairy herd was decimated by a PBB contamination. The cattle were seriously ill for eight months before Rick Halbert and his consultants finally discovered that the herd's health problems were the result of a PBB contamination of their feed. During that period, Rick Halbert spent all of his time attempting to discover the source of his herd's problems, ignoring his family and becoming increasingly withdrawn.[18]

Halbert's obsession grew out of his immersion in a situation that was simultaneously hopeful and hopeless. It was hopeless in the sense that his herd's health was deteriorating in front of his eyes, and that the causes of that deterioration were indecipherable to both himself and his cadre of experts. However, he believed that it was still possible to find the source of his problem and to save his herd. In his own mind, he just had to ask the right questions and look in the right place. As a result, finding the source of the problem became an immense preoccupation for Rick Halbert.

Levine reports a similar response to the Love Canal contamination. The residents of the Love Canal area had lived with the toxic waste dump site for a long time, in some cases more than twenty years. Concern about the canal had been historically sporadic and had centered around specific issues, such as the discovery of tarry substances in residential sump pumps, the spontaneous appearance of toxic sink holes in the neighborhood, and the insistent presence of chemical odors. Concerns about the canal became more urgent when the authorities began to publicly announce their concerns about the dump site. Many neighborhood residents became vigilant—seeking out information about the canal and wondering if it had been the cause of the many unexplained and persistent health problems which they had experienced over the years. Their worst fears seem to be confirmed when the New York State Health Commissioner recommended that pregnant women and children under age two move out of the area.[19] When Love Canal residents heard the announcement, they "ran out into the neighborhood streets and were united in a moment of real panic."[20]

The mood of panic, fear, and deep concern persisted as Love Canal residents realized that they had been unwittingly living in a dangerous situation for years. They began to realize that their situation was, in a sense, hopeless, because they had probably been injured already by the chemicals in the canal. At the same time, they understood that their situation was not entirely beyond their control, because they still had the option of moving and in so doing stopping further toxic exposures. Unfortunately, evacuation was an expensive proposition, and financial assistance was contingent on the results of scientific studies of the health effects of the dump site.

Thus Love Canal residents had two incentives for being vigilant about the health effects of the canal: (1) to protect themselves from both past and ongoing toxic exposures and (2) to make certain that the government did accurate and honest studies of the health effects of the canal. As a result, an exceedingly vigilant pattern of information-seeking behavior appeared in the majority of the Love Canal area residents.[21]

The residents of Love Canal believed in the scientific process. They believed that if the correct studies were done, they would be able to move; and they believed that the involved governments would keep their word in this regard. But after the White House refused relocation assistance in spite of an EPA study showing abnormal chromosomal damage in residents surveyed, anger and panic prevailed at Love Canal. Two EPA employees were seized and held hostage for several hours at the Love Canal Homeowners Association office. For area residents, the possibilities of protecting themselves from the ongoing dangers posed by the canal seemed once again out of reach.

Hypervigilant preoccupation has been found in other situations involving an invisible contamination. Atomic veterans who believe that they have been injured by radiation await, with dread, each new symptom. They have lived, and continue to live, in fear that each new symptom will be the one that takes them to their physician to find out that they have cancer or some other terminal illness. In response to this fear and in response to having medical conditions that their physicians could not explain, diagnose, or treat, veterans have searched in desperation for physicians who would understand and be able to help. It has not been unusual for an atomic veteran to consult with ten, sometimes even twenty, physicians in the search for diagnosis and treatment for his symptoms. An atomic veteran named John, whose neurological problems were eventually diagnosed as dermatomyositis, reports that he used to call his doctor the very first moment he noticed a new symptom, although he was convinced that he was going to die anyway.[22] For this man, and others like him, the paradox of hypervigilance is that, on the one hand, this veteran assumes the worst: "I thought every new symptom meant I was going to die," but on the other hand, he still believes that he can help himself, and he has continued to seek the help of physicians.

The hypervigilant response to the invisible contaminations is part of yet another pattern of response to these exposures. In chapter 5 we saw that the

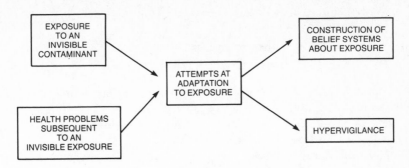

Figure 12–1. Adaptational Sequence (#2)

attempt to adapt to an invisible exposure can generate an unwanted wealth of experienced uncertainties and adaptational dilemmas. It is now becoming evident that further attempts at adaptation generate a characteristic cognitive and behavioral response to that exposure. Individuals exposed to an invisible environmental contaminant also: (1) construct belief systems about the nature of that exposure as a means of appraising it, and (2) adopt a hypervigilant response to that exposure as a means of protecting themselves from the threats that it poses for them. This later sequence of events can be diagrammed as shown in figure 12–1.

The Causes of Hypervigilance

At the center of Janis's conflict theory model is an articulation of the "subjective beliefs" or "mediating psychological conditions" that give rise to each of the separate patterns of stress response. For example, the single belief that both galvanizes and mediates the pattern of unconflicted inertia is the belief that there is "no serious risk from the current course of action."[23] Janis is interested in the cognitive conditions, or beliefs, that generate each pattern of response to threat because he is, once again, interested in learning what conditions foster vigilance and how they differ from those that underlie each of the four defective coping patterns.[24] He is interested in learning how to promote vigilance in both disaster and in crucial decision-making situations.

The conflict theory model posits that the hypervigilant pattern of response is generated when the respondent simultaneously holds four beliefs about a particular threatening situation (for example, a fire in a crowded movie theater). The beliefs are as follows:[25]

1. Adherence to the current course of action [continuing to watch the movie] will result in serious risk.

2. Adherence to a new course of action [fleeing through the only visible exit] will also result in serious risk.
3. A better solution to the problem can be found.
4. There is insufficient time to search for and evaluate a better solution.

If a person holds beliefs one and two in a threatening situation, but believes that no better solution can be found, that person will, according to Janis's model, adopt a defensive avoidance response. In so doing, that person will avoid making a successful adaptation to the threat.

Janis and Mann[26] have diagrammed the sequential sets of conditions that give rise to the various patterns of response to threat. These are shown in figure 12–2.

The conditions that breed the hypervigilant response are the simultaneous beliefs that one is at serious risk, that a better response to the threat is somehow available, but that time is not sufficient to determine what that better response is. Thus, a paradoxical appraisal of a threatening situation lies at the heart of the hypervigilant response. The threatened person believes that: (1) a potentially successful response to a serious threat is possible, but also believes that (2) it is not likely that they will be able to find this successful response.

In Janis's formulation, this second belief develops because the threatened person does not have sufficient time to find the successful response. As we have already seen, hypervigilance can also occur in situations in which time is not an issue. It can occur in protracted situations of threat in which the problem is one of insufficient *information* to permit successful appraisal of the threat at hand. This was the case in the Brighton gas explosion disaster cited by Janis, and in all of the other invisible exposures considered above.

Therefore, I would like to suggest a slight modification of the mediating conditions, or beliefs, of hypervigilance as articulated by Janis. I would change the fourth of his mediating beliefs, and do so not because I think it incorrect, but because it can be expanded to be more inclusive.

From our review of the conditions in which hypervigilance has been found to occur, it would seem that the fourth condition for hypervigilance can be more correctly stated as: escape from the threatening situation seems impossible to the threatened person because there is either insufficient time or insufficient information with which to master that threat. Such is the situation faced by both the atomic veteran who has been harmed by radiation, and the theater occupant who does not have sufficient time to consider his escape options in a burning theater.

To believe that successful escape from a threatening situation is impossible is to believe that mastery of that situation is impossible. This fourth belief is the distinctive condition that gives rise to hypervigilance. As Janis has shown, if the threatened person believes that "sufficient time to search for

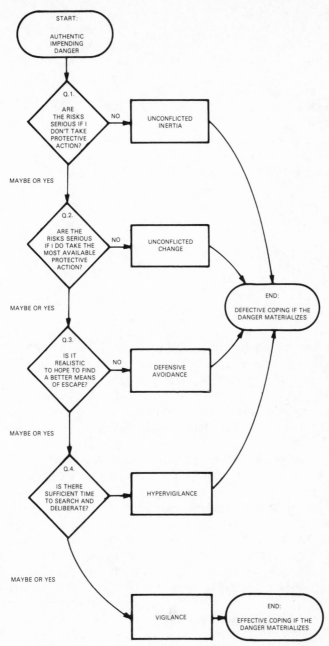

Source: I.L. Janis and L. Mann, *Decision Making: A Psychological Analysis of Conflict, Choice and Commitment* (New York: The Free Press, 1977).

Figure 12–2. The Conflict Theory Model

and evaluate a better solution" is available,[27] if that person believes that mastery of the imminent threat is indeed possible, a vigilant pattern of response will be the result. Both the vigilant and hypervigilant respondent believe that a means of mastering a threatening situation exists, but only the vigilant person believes that he or she will actually be able to discover and implement that means of mastery.

Contrasting the conditions necessary for hypervigilance with conditions that generate learned helplessness is also instructive. Consideration of the difference between these two responses to threat points out the causal role of the paradoxical threat appraisal that lies at the heart of the hypervigilant response pattern. The hypervigilant individual believes, simultaneously, that escape from a threatening situation is both possible and impossible. In learned helplessness, the threatened subject believes only that escape is not possible. Learned helplessness can be seen as a sixth type of response to a threatening situation. It is characterized by total and abject surrender to the occurrence of inevitable noxious events. The subject who has learned to be helpless totally gives up trying to alter threatening or harmful circumstances.[28]

In distinct contrast, the hypervigilant person becomes preoccupied with escaping from the threat in question.

The psychological condition of the hypervigilant response seems, then, to be the realization that, even though mastery of a threatening situation is possible, it is not likely to be achieved. In the case of a fire in a crowded theater or a tornado warning received seconds before the tornado strikes, mastery is not possible because sufficient time to evaluate and respond to the situation is not available. In the case of an invisible exposure, mastery is not possible because the information necessary to appraise and cope with the situation successfully is not available.

The person who has been exposed to radiation soon learns that nothing can be done about a potential cancer until it becomes clinically apparent. The people being exposed to toxic chemicals at Love Canal could not adapt to that exposure because they did not learn of its existence until it had already been going on for years. Clearly, mastery of the threats posed by the invisible exposures prove to be an elusive, if not impossible, task.

Eventually, the exposed person learns that medical science will be unable to help him protect himself from the health effects of the contaminant to which he has been exposed. He learns that he will just have to wait and see, and that there is no way he can empirically cope with and master the threats posed to his health by the exposure. At this juncture, the exposed person has two equally unattractive options. Either he can choose to forget—or deny—the possibility that his health has been compromised, or he can continue to attempt to pursue a vigilant course.

For many of the people who have been exposed to an invisible contaminant, dismissal or denial of the threats posed by an exposure is neither a desirable nor a possible option. Such people attempt to remain vigilant about the medical and environmental threats posed to their health by a past or ongoing exposure. As in other circumstances in which ambiguity of threat renders mastery of that threat impossible, vigilance becomes hypervigilance. Continued lack of mastery leads to fixation, and vigilance escalates into an almost total preoccupation with the health effects of an invisible exposure. Hypervigilance will emerge as a prominent mode of response to an exposure as the exposed person discovers that the pursuit of vigilance is not leading to mastery of his or her situation. If hypervigilance persists and becomes the basis of a fixation, it can become the nidus of a traumatic neurosis. We will be taking a closer look at the hypervigilant response to an invisible contamination in chapters 14 and 16.

13
Traumatic Neurosis

In the second half of the nineteenth century a number of clinicians became concerned with tracking down the psychological etiology of the neuroses. The term *neurosis* was first used to designate a diagnostic category in the writings of the Scottish physician William Cullen in the middle of the eighteenth century. Cullen coined the term as a replacement for the then-current designation "nervous diseases," a diagnostic category developed and used by the British physicians Thomas Willis and Thomas Sydenham. Both Willis and Sydenham regarded nervous diseases as diseases caused by disturbances in the functioning of the central nervous system.

Cullen used the term neurosis in much the same manner that Willis and Sydenman used the term nervous disorder. Neuroses, Cullen said, are "all those preternatural affections of sense and motion without pyrexia . . . and all those that do not depend upon a topical affection of the organs, but upon a more general affection of the nervous system and those powers of the system."[1] The central distinction that Cullen was trying to make is that the neuroses should be regarded as those illnesses caused by a dysfunction of the nervous system, as opposed to the dysfunction of a particular bodily organ.

Cullen also said that "the term neurosis should be used to refer only to diseases originating from direct alterations of the nervous system."[2] He believed that the neuroses were due to definite decay, either of the intellect or of the voluntary or involuntary nervous system.[3] In Cullen's estimation, the disease category of neurosis included paralysis, syncope, hypochondria, tetanus, epilepsy, asthma, whooping cough, diabetes, hysteria, melancholia, and mania. Cullen's list is a rather far-ranging one, and it differs considerably from our contemporary notions of the diagnostic entities designated by the term neurosis. However, a rather comtemporary critique of the then-clinical usage of the term neurosis was made by the eighteenth-century physician Robert Whytt, who wrote, "It is often said that physicians have bestowed the term nervous on all of those disorders whose nature and causes they were ignorant of."[4]

Closer inspection of Cullen's conception of the nervous system leads one to conclude, however, that in an important sense he used the term neurosis in much the same manner that it is being used in the twentieth century. Through his creation of the diagnostic category of the neuroses Cullen articulated the position that there exists a group of illnesses whose causes we would today call psychological. He didn't put the case in exactly those words, but a careful look at his conception of the nervous system indicates that this is really the essence of his position.

Cullen saw the nervous system as "the instrument of the anima." He saw the nervous system as the physical substance through which a person's soul energizes and gives life to the body. He believed that the tone and irritability found in the solid parts of the body, which he regarded as the primary manifestations of life, are transmitted to the body by the nervous system, in the form of a fluid similar to ether.

Thus Cullen regarded the nervous system as being the material medium in which the soul operated and imparted life to the body. In positing the existence of a category of diseases caused by nervous system dysfunction, Cullen was actually positing the existence of a category of diseases caused by disorders of the soul, which today we call diseases of the mind.

This derivative Cartesian conception of the nervous system and of illness was not unique in this time to Cullen. In fact, his position is rather representative of the thinking of his period. Similar conceptions had been previously held by both Sydenham and Willis. Georg Ernst Stahl, the influential eighteenth-century physician and chemist, held that "the chemical and physical reactions of the body are kept going only by means of the soul."[5] Each of these men adhered to a conception of soul and central nervous system that can only be described as an amalgam of metaphysical monism and ontological dualism; a conception in which two entities, soul and nervous system, are present in one substance, the material tissue of the nervous system.

In proposing the existence of the neuroses, Cullen posited the existence of a diagnostic category of illnesses that had in common a particular etiology. This category was made up of diseases caused by dysfunction of the nervous system; as we have seen, this also meant dysfunction of the soul or mind. Cullen's diagnostic category of the neuroses was not restricted to diseases that manifest as somatic symptoms. The neuroses included diseases that could become symptomatic as somatic, behavioral, cognitive, and emotional symptoms. Thus Cullen's category of neurosis embodied our contemporary notion that psychological phenomena can cause both somatic and mental illness. Cullen's conception of the neuroses was the most influential of his time, and was adopted, for example, by the French physician-psychiatrist Philippe Pinel.

During the course of the nineteenth century, the long list of diseases considered to be caused by nervous system dysfunction was gradually reduced until by the end of the century only a very few diseases were still thought to be neuroses. This change was the immediate and conscious result of the appearance and rapid ascendance of the anatomoclinical paradigm in medicine. The anatomoclinical paradigm, which completely transformed medicine and made it into the discipline that it is today, holds that diseases are caused by localized anatomopathological lesions. The symptoms of a disease are caused by diseased tissue. Pneumonia is a microbial infection of the lung. Cirrhosis is a scarring of the liver. Subarachnoid hemorrhage is the rupture of a cerebral artery, usually in the Circle of Willis at the base of the brain.

In our own time, it is hard to imagine that the practice of medicine could have ever occurred outside of the anatomoclinical paradigm, but prior to its emergence the symptom, as opposed to the pathological lesion, was the central organizing principle of medicine. Disease entities were defined, diagnosed, and treated in terms of symptoms. The confusion that this approach is capable of generating can still be appreciated today within the field of psychiatry. In contemporary psychiatry, diagnostic entities are still defined in terms of their symptoms. The psychological equivalent of the anatomopathological lesion has yet to be agreed upon within the field, and the result is the confused field that is our contemporary form of psychiatry. (It is my position that the psychological equivalent of the anatomopathological lesion is the fixation. However, thorough presentation of the case for this position is too lengthy a tangent for this book and will be presented in a forthcoming book entitled *Fixation: The Reorganization of Psychiatry.*)

With the advent of the anatomoclinical paradigm, physicians began a systematic search for the anatomopathological lesions causing all known diseases. This search led to a contraction of the list of diseases that were thought of as being neuroses. If a disease that had once been considered to be a neurosis was found to be caused by a particular pathological lesion, it could, of course, no longer be regarded as a neurosis. The neuroses were still thought of as generalized functionalized disorders of the nervous system. Thus the model of disease presented in the anatomoclinical paradigm was, and is, in direct conflict with the conception of nervous disease, or neurosis. With the ascendancy of the anatomoclinical paradigm, nineteenth-century physicians generally came to believe that it would only be a matter of time until the discovery of pathological lesions would entirely eliminate the diagnostic category of the neuroses. They believed that causal pathological lesions would be found for all of the neuroses.

They were almost correct. Toward the end of the nineteenth century, the spectrum of somatic illnesses still considered to be neuroses had dwindled down to a few elusive diseases. Of the remaining illnesses still identified as neuroses, hysteria was the diagnostic entity that received the most attention. Hysteria was regarded as being of central theoretical import because it seemed possible to many physicians that it was not caused by somatic lesions as predicted by the anatomoclinical paradigm. As a result, many important physicians of the era turned their attention to the problem of determining its cause. Among them were Moritz Benedikt, Jean Martin Charcot, Josef Breuer, Pierre Janet, and Sigmund Freud.

During this same period, and in response to the appearance of the anatomoclinical paradigm, the concept of neurosis went through several changes. It was changed by its defenders in their attempts to somehow integrate the notion of neurosis with the truth contained within the new paradigm. For example, the French physician Archille-Louis Foville defined neuroses as diseases that were anatomically localized in the nervous system, but somehow not caused by an anatomical alteration of the nervous system. This was just one of several definitions of neurosis that appeared in the first half of the nineteenth century as attempts to: (1) preserve the notion that there is a category of illnesses caused by psychological phenomena and (2) integrate this notion with the idea that diseases are caused by localized anatomical lesions.

Despite this movement in the definition of the neuroses toward a position of consistency with the anatomoclinical paradigm, a number of people continued to be interested in the psychological causes of the neuroses in general and of hysteria in particular. As if in some way impelled by the cultural milieu of late nineteenth-century Europe, a number of physicians became almost simultaneously interested in the role of fixations, or fixed ideas, in the etiology of hysteria. The basic concept of the fixed idea is that neurotic symptoms are caused by the repressed mental representation of a particular experience. This repressed representation is the fixed idea, and it is thought that the symptoms of a neurosis are a symbolic expression of the notions of reality contained in the fixed idea.

Moritz Benedikt, a Viennese neurologist, was the first physician to present any systematic thoughts on the role of fixation in the causation of hysteria. "In a series of publications that appeared between the years of 1864 and 1895 Benedikt showed that the cause of many cases of both hysteria and the other neuroses resided in a painful secret, mostly pertaining to sexual life, and that many patients could be cured by the confession of their pathogenic secrets."[6] In 1885 the French physician Charcot took this exposition a step further by providing dramatic experimental proof that a fixed idea could cause a somatic symptom. In a series of brilliant experiments, he demonstrated that the clinical equivalent of a traumatic paralysis of the arm could be induced in a subject by means of a posthypnotic suggestion.

A traumatic paralysis is a paralysis that develops subsequent to a traumatic experience (for example, a railway accident) but for which no neurological lesion can be found. In other words, no physical explanation can be found for the paralysis. Charcot began his experiments by demonstrating that the symptoms of the naturally occurring traumatic paralyses are characteristically different from the symptoms of the organic paralyses—those for which an organic lesion could be found. Then he induced paralysis of the arm in several experimental subjects by means of posthypnotic suggestion. He demonstrated that the symptoms of the hypnotically induced paralysis were identical to the symptoms of the spontaneously occurring traumatic paralysis. Finally, he demonstrated that the symptoms of the spontaneously occurring hysterical paralyses had the same characteristics as the traumatic and hypnotically induced paralyses. "Charcot and his auditors considered that these demonstrations provided scientific proof of the psychogenesis of the traumatic paralyses."[7] At the very least, these experiments seem to demonstrate that an unconscious fixed idea can cause a somatic symptom.

Breuer and Freud took the next step and demonstrated that, in addition to causing traumatic paralyses, fixed unconscious ideas could also be the cause of the psychological symptoms of hysteria.[8] In 1888 the German psychiatrist Paul Moebius had defined hysteria as "morbid changes in the body that are caused by [mental] representations."[9] Breuer and Freud contended in their 1893 paper that the entire spectrum of hysterical symptoms, including the psychological symptoms, are caused by the fixed ideas that result from psychological trauma. Their theory was that the traumatic experience is excluded from consciousness and consequently becomes, as a fixed unconscious idea, the cause of the hysterical symptom or symptoms. The memory of the traumatic experience was thought to be expressed in symbolic fashion as the psychological symptoms of an hysterical illness.

In 1896 Freud published a paper entitled "The Heredity and Etiology of the Neuroses." In it he contended that all of the neuroses, and not just hysteria, were caused by unconscious fixed ideas generated by the intentional forgetting of traumatic experiences. To embody this extension of his theory, he proposed a new classification of the neuroses, each of which he considered to be caused by a specific type of sexual trauma. He recognized at that point four types of neurosis. They are listed below with the trauma that he regarded as their causes:

1. Neurasthenia: masturbation
2. Anxiety neurosis: frustrated sexual stimulation
3. Hysteria: Sexual abuse by an adult passively suffered in childhood
4. Obsessional Neurosis: Sexual abuse by an adult that was enjoyed by the child.

Pierre Janet, the French philosopher and physician, also put forth a theory based on his own clinical experience that directly implicated fixed subconscious ideas as the cause of neurosis. He produced a number of case studies that provide graphic demonstration of the fact that unconscious fixed ideas can and do cause the symptoms of the neuroses. He disagreed, however, with Freud's notion that the contents of these fixed ideas must of necessity involve sexual material. Carl Jung, at a later time and in a different way, took much the same position. Jung's concept of fixation is embodied in his notion of the complex.

Freud eventually discarded his traumatic theory of neurosogenesis and adopted a different type of fixation theory of the etiology of the neuroses. This second theory is the well-known psychosexual stage theory, in which neurosis is depicted as being caused by a fixation to one of the infantile stages of psychosexual development. With the advent of this second model, the role of fixed ideas or images in the etiology of the neuroses was more or less discarded by psychiatrists.

There has been, since that time, one exception to this generic trend in the field of psychiatry: it is still generally held that the traumatic neuroses, or posttraumatic stress disorders as they are now called, are caused by a fixation to a mental representation of a traumatic experience. There continues to be considerable debate as to whether this traumatic fixation occurs because of the existence of a character predisposition, or latent neurosis, on the part of the patient, or because of the nature of the traumatic event itself.[10] However, there is no question that the consequent neurosis is both mediated by and caused by a fixation to a representation of a traumatic event.

Freud himself was puzzled by the traumatic neuroses and their obvious relationship to traumatic experiences. The analysis of these neuroses seems to have led him on numerous occasions to reconsider the importance of the role of trauma in the etiology of the neuroses.[11] One such occasion was World War I, which forced Freud to grapple with the then-prevalent phenomenon of shell shock.[12] However, the psychosexual stage theory always managed to endure the questions generated by the traumatic neuroses.

Traumatic neurosis is a condition that occurs to some people who have been through a major traumatic experience. The traumatic neuroses have been found to occur in persons who have experienced military combat,[13] internment in Nazi concentration camps,[14] nuclear holocaust,[15] rape,[16] the death of a spouse,[17] railway accidents,[18] and the like. Traumatic neurosis has been recognized as a clinical entity since the seventeenth century,[19] but today the American Psychiatric Association uses the term posttraumatic stress disorder to refer to this entity.[20] The symptoms of posttraumatic stress disorder are as follows:

1. Reexperiencing the traumatic event by:
   (a) Recurrent and intrusive recollections of the event,
   (b) Recurrent dreams of the event,
   (c) Suddenly acting or feeling as if the traumatic event were occurring because of an association with an environmental or ideational stimulus.

2. Numbing of responsiveness to, or involvement with, the external world, beginning some time after the traumatic event(s) as shown by either:
    (a) Markedly diminished interest in one or more significant activities,
    (b) Feelings of detachment or estrangement from others, or
    (c) Marked constriction of affective responses.

3. At least two of the following (not present prior to traumatic event):
    (a) Hyperalertness or exaggerated startle response,
    (b) Initial, middle, or terminal sleep disturbance,
    (c) Guilt about surviving when others have not, or about behavior required to achieve survival,
    (d) Memory impairment or trouble concentrating,
    (e) Avoidance of activities that arouse recollection of traumatic event, and
    (f) Intensification of symptoms by exposure to events that symbolize or resemble the traumatic event.

These symptoms may or may not be accompanied by functional neurological symptoms.[21] Horowitz, as we shall be seeing, has stressed the oscillating biphasic nature of the symptoms of posttraumatic stress disorder.[22]

In discussing the causes of posttraumatic stress disorder, it is useful to remember that two types of events cause this entity to develop: (1) traumatic environmental events and (2) psychological events. Causally, they are related as independent variable and intervening variable. This relationship can be diagrammed as shown in figure 13–1. In other words, a traumatic environmental event causes a structural change in the mind of the traumatized person that results in the development of the symptoms of a traumatic neurosis. Much theoretical confusion has resulted from the fact that the same event can have different effects on different people. A harmful event may cause one person to develop a traumatic neurosis, while another person who experienced the same event may have no psychological aftereffects at all.

The structural or psychological essence of posttraumatic stress disorder is that the affected person continues to live as though a previous traumatic event is still occurring. The traumatized person continues to live, to varying degrees, in the images of self and world created by that traumatic experience. In other words, the traumatized person is fixated to those images. Recent

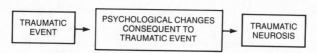

Figure 13–1. The Pathogenesis of Traumatic Neurosis (#1)

history provides us with the example of the Vietnam War veterans who came home to the United States but continued to live, in their minds, in the violent jungles of Vietnam.

Freud was the first person to link the phenomenon of fixation to the occurrence of the traumatic neurosis per se. In his 1916–1917 lecture series,[23] he said that "the traumatic neuroses give a clear indication that fixation to the moment of the traumatic accident lies at their root." He went on to say that "it is as though these patients are not finished with the traumatic situation, as though they were still faced by it as an immediate task which had not been dealt with."

Kardiner, in consequence of his work on the traumatic neuroses of World War II, also found fixation to the traumatic event to be at the center of the traumatic neurosis. Kardiner saw traumatic neurosis as a form of ego contraction, in which a person loses many of his or her previously developed modes of relating to the world. He saw this contraction in ego capacity as a consequence of the traumatized person's fixation to the traumatic event. As a result of this fixation, the traumatized soldier becomes a very literal version of the person he was at the time of the traumatic event.

Kardiner found, for example, traumatized soldiers whose neurotic symptoms included either a repetitive tic or a repetitive and ritualized form of behavior. In Kardiner's words, "the subject acts as if the original traumatic situation was still in existence and engages in protective devices which failed on the original occasion. This means in effect that his conception of the outer world and conception of himself and his resources have been permanently altered."[24] Kardiner also goes on to state that such an individual gives evidence of being "in a continuous state of heightened vigilance."[25]

Kardiner also finds evidence of fixation to the traumatic event in victims' "hallucinatory reproductions of sensations originally experienced in the traumatic event. In this instance the symptom contains the idea 'I am still living in the traumatic situation.'"[26] He also finds the lingering effects of fixation in motor disturbances, repetitive dreams that reproduce the traumatic event and syncopal episodes provoked by "external stimuli which resemble the occasion of [an] original loss of consciousness."[27]

Horowitz takes the similar position (rendered in terms of cognitive theory) that traumatized patients continue to live in the memory of the traumatic event because the images of self and world contained in that event cannot be integrated into that person's previous images of self and world. In Horowitz's words, "completion of [cognitive processing] involves the resolution of differences between new information and enduring schemata. . . . A familiar non-stressful event is likely to be quickly and automatically assimilated. Completion of cognitive processing will occur and the information in active memory storage will be rapidly terminated. The information in novel and stressful events, however, can not be rapidly processed. The point of relative completion is not achieved and so termination of active memory retention does not occur."[28]

In other words, because the cognitive processing of a traumatic event cannot be rapidly completed, the memory of that event remains in a form of information storage that Horowitz calls active memory. The retention of this representation of a traumatic event in active memory is Horowitz's rendering of the concept of fixation, and is seen as the cause of the symptoms of posttraumatic stress disorder in his model.[29] Within this model, the symptoms of posttraumatic stress disorder are seen as an expression of the processes by which the traumatized person's mind attempts to integrate the meanings of the traumatic event into the images of self and world held prior to the traumatic event.

Horowitz postulates that the repetitive and compulsive representation of the traumatic event in consciousness occurs as a result of this fixation in active memory. These repetitive representations of the traumatic event are what Horowitz calls the intrusive symptoms of posttraumatic stress disorder. The intrusive symptoms are the often-documented reexperiencing of a traumatic event that occurs to the traumatized person. This reexperiencing of a traumatic event occurs in the form of stereotypical dreams and nightmares, repetitive thoughts and images of the event, rumination, hallucination, and repetitive ritual reenactments of the event. These symptoms occur during what Horowitz calls the intrusion phase of posttraumatic stress disorder. He sees the intrusive symptoms of this neurosis as a part of the process by which the traumatized person's mind actively attempts to assimilate the unintegrated representation of a traumatic event.

Horowitz calls the second basic phase of posttraumatic stress disorder symptomatology the denial phase. During this phase, memories of the traumatic event are successfully warded off by the traumatized person's ego, and cognitive processing of the traumatic event temporarily ceases. During the denial phase, intrusive symptoms do not occur. The primary symptoms of this phase are emotional numbing, ideational avoidance, and behavioral constriction. The general course of posttraumatic stress disorder is one in which periods of intrusive symptoms alternate, or oscillate, with periods of denial symptoms.

Given, then, that a fixation to the images of world and self contained in a traumatic event is the psychological lesion, if you will, that causes the development of the symptoms of the traumatic neuroses, what are the situational factors that cause such a fixation to develop? Fixation seems to occur to a person in consequence of being involved in a situation in which that person does not master a threatening event. Traumatic neuroses develop, for example, in the person who by virtue of being in prolonged combat is under constant threat and by virtue of the nature of that situation is unable to eliminate the threat posed to his life by the enemy soldiers.

This inability to master threat was in particular evidence during the Vietnam War, and was a consequence of the conditions faced by American combatants.

The psychologist Victor DeFazio has noted that the Vietnam War was a "conflict fought against an indigenous revolutionary army. This fact is important because it accounts for the very special character of the war. Its clandestine nature led to considerable brutalization on both sides. It left American troops with a sense of helplessness at not being able to confront the enemy in set-piece battles." The threat posed by the enemy was such that the more or less conventional rules of warfare broke down. American soldiers were in situations in which they could be attacked in a way and at any time, which made mastery of the threat posed by the enemy a full time and difficult affair. "The spectre of being shot at and having friends killed and maimed by virtually unseen forces generated considerable rage which came to be displaced on anyone or anything available."[30]

The inability of victims to master a threatening event is the condition that leads to a fixation to that event. To quote, again, this telling passage from Freud, "it is as though these patients are not finished with the traumatic situation, as though they were still faced by it as an immediate task which had not been dealt with."[31] Because the traumatized person does not finish the task of protecting him- or herself from the traumatic event, he or she remains fixated to that event and continues to try to master it. Herein lies the basis of fixation. The Vietnam veteran continues to protect himself from the dangers of the jungle even though he has returned to the United States.[32] Traumatized nuclear holocaust victims live as though they are already dead; killed by the atomic bomb that they actually survived.[33] The victim of rape lives in fear of future rape.[34]

Kardiner defined a traumatic event as "an external influence necessitating an abrupt change in adaptation which the organism fails to meet.[35] He also found that "the traumatic event creates excitations beyond the possibility of mastering, inflicting a severe blow to the total ego organization."[36] To Kardiner's eye, this lack of mastery at the time of trauma persists within the mind of the traumatized person:

> Some portion of the integrated ego is either destroyed or inhibited; a portion which normally enables the individual to carry out certain actions automatically on the basis of innumerable successes in the past. This portion of the ego is injured in the traumatic experience, and what results is an inhibition. This portion of the ego has, moreover, a protective influence on the ego; these protective maneuvers we call mastery or adaptation. Being deserted by these protective devices . . . the subjects feel deserted and obliged to face a world that must annihilate him because he no longer has any defense against it.[37]

A traumatic event, then, is an event in which a person feels helpless because mastery of that event is not possible. Freud said that "the essence of a traumatic situation is an experience of helplessness on the part of the ego in the face of [an] accumulation of excitation, whether of internal or external origin."[38] Furst has come to much the same conclusion: "The psychic content of the trauma is explicit: it involves the feeling of helplessness in the face of overwhelming danger."[39] Perhaps, and I say only perhaps, it is this sense of helplessness that makes it impossible for the traumatized mind to assimilate the traumatic event.

In addition, the lack of mastery that occurs in the face of a truly traumatic event often leads the traumatized person to lose his or her sense of invulnerability to danger. It seems that, for most people, the pursuit of life involves the adoption of the belief that one is invulnerable and capable of mastering all threat.[40] In Horowitz's words, the "expectation of personal omnipotence or total control is unrealistic, but it is nonetheless a universal hope and sometimes a deeply felt personal belief. The failure to prevent a stress event such as an accident is regarded as a loss of control and conflicts with the wish to have power and mastery."[41]

Evidence of the central role that the lack of mastery of a traumatic event plays in causing a traumatic neurosis can be found in the nature of the symptoms of the resulting neurosis. In Furst's words, "In trauma, one often finds . . . that the resultant symptom represents a belated attempt to master the underlying trauma or group of traumas."[42] Furst explains that "dynamically, the experience of being traumatized confronts the ego with the task of belatedly mastering the overwhelming stimulus and its immediate repercussions. One manifestation of the struggle for mastery is the posttraumatic anxiety dream, in which the trauma is reexperienced, either nakedly or in a disguised way, and psychically repeated in milder forms. Another manifestation involves the reliving of the trauma in waking life."[43] For example, the traumatized soldier might have repetitive dreams of the time the enemy overran his position killing everyone but himself. The rape victim might mentally reexperience her rape while walking alone at night.

Freud, himself, was of the opinion that recurring traumatic dreams were an attempt to master the original situation.[44] Sandler writes that "the bulk of the material that the patients bring to analysis leads in one way or another back to the traumatic episode. The memory of it has remained as a dangerous unassimilated drive cathected experience that can only be dealt with by massive repression, or if this fails, by attempts at mastery through repetition."[45]

Once the original event has passed, the arena of attempted mastery shifts from the physical locus of the traumatic event to the mind of the traumatized person. Here the traumatized person attempts to rework, or recomprehend, the experience. The goal of reworking the cognitive representation of the traumatic event is to render it into a form that can be assimilated into the person's pretraumatic images of world and self. In Horowitz's words,

> After a traumatic event, there is a compulsive tendency toward repetition of some aspects of the experience. . . . These repetitions may occur in spite of pronounced conscious efforts at avoidance and suppression but are not necessarily static replicas of the original experience. A series of successive revisions in content and form are frequently noted in clinical studies. Often, such repetitions may eventually lose their intrusive and involuntary nature. The change in content and reduced intrusiveness indicates that a progressive mastery of the experience has taken place.[46]

In summary, then, three basic conclusions can be reached about the etiology of posttraumatic stress disorder, or traumatic neurosis: (1) the traumatic neuroses are caused when a traumatic event initiates a change in the structure of the traumatized person's mind that produces the symptoms of the neurosis, (2) the pathogenic structural change caused by the traumatic event is a fixation, in active memory, to the images of world and self contained in that event, and (3) the traumatic event is a significant and threatening event, which the traumatized person is unable to master. The causal sequence implied by this analysis can be schematically summarized as shown in figure 13–2.

It appears that a similar sequence of events can occur in consequence of an exposure to an invisible environmental contaminant. The similarity begins with the fact that achieving mastery over the threats posed by an exposure to an invisible contaminant is virtually impossible. Mastery is impossible, as we have already seen, because of the environmental and medical invisibility of these contaminants. The invisibility makes it impossible for exposed persons to obtain the information that they need to successfully appraise and master the threatening situation created by an invisible exposure.

In different traumatic situations, there can be variations in the time that it takes for people to realize that they won't be able to master the threatening event. In an acute traumatic event, for example a tornado, it bcomes apparent almost immediately that mastery of the situation will not be possible. The same can also be said about rape, an airplane crash, or warfare—although in war the experience of helplessness may be protracted.

The situation is somewhat different with the invisible environmental contaminants. Most often, it is not immediately evident to the exposed person

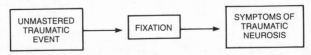

Figure 13–2. The Pathogenesis of Traumatic Neurosis (#2)

that mastery of the exposure and its consequences will not be possible. This difficulty in accurately assessing the prospects of mastery may occur for any number of reasons in an invisible exposure.

Among many other possibilities, it may not be immediately apparent that mastery is not possible because the exposed person may not even be aware that exposure to an invisible contaminant is taking place. It may happen because the exposed person doesn't know how large a dose of contaminant he or she has received. Or it may be that the contaminant has a latency period, and the exposed person doesn't know for certain whether he or she has been physically injured by an exposure that has already occurred. A number of other reasons related to the invisible nature of the involved contaminant may also work to prevent the exposed person from realizing that mastery of this threat will not be possible.

As we have already seen, it is only in the process of attempting to cope with an invisible exposure that a person learns how difficult it is to master the threats posed by that exposure. It is only in the process of attempting to adapt to and master an invisible exposure that a person begins to learn that the information needed to make that adaptation is not available.

For these reasons, then, it generally takes the person exposed to an invisible contaminant a longer period of time than the victims of an acute trauma to understand that mastery of their situation will not be possible. Nonetheless, the psychological effects of an exposure to an invisible contaminant can be much the same as those of an immediate and palpable trauma. They are the same in the sense that the person exposed to an invisible contaminant often develops a fixation to the exposure. The fixation occurs for much the same reason that it does in an acute trauma: the exposed person comes to realize that he or she will not be able to master the medical threats posed by the exposure. The traumatized soldier remains fixated to the Vietnamese jungle in an attempt to gain cognitive mastery over the events that overwhelmed him there. The person exposed to an invisible contaminant remains vigilantly fixated to the exposure as a means of attempting to gain mastery over its still-unfolding health effects.

The fixation of the person exposed to an invisible environmental contaminant takes a different form from the fixation of the person caught up in an acute trauma. The psychological fixation that occurs to an acute traumatic event, for example, a rape or a nuclear bomb explosion, is a fixation to the images of world and self contained in the traumatic event. The traumatized person continues to live, long after the occurrence of that trauma, within the world portrayed by the imagery of that event. Fixation to that imagery occurs at the time of that event, and this fixation will usually manifest as the symptoms of a traumatic neurosis either immediately or within months.

The psychological fixation caused by an invisible exposure is, at root, a fixation to the belief that one has endured a dangerous exposure. Eventually this belief develops into a secondary fixation to the behaviors adopted by an exposed person to protect himself or herself from the consequences of that exposure. Mere adoption of this belief and the resultant protective behavior is not in and of itself a fixation. The determination that an invisible exposure has been dangerous usually begins innocently enough, as the cognitive ground on which a vigilant response to that exposure is based. It can be simply the appraisal adopted by the person who decides that it is necessary to protect himself or herself from the health effects of an exposure to an invisible environmental contaminant.

The belief that an invisible exposure has been dangerous can become the core of a much larger cognitive and behavioral fixation as the exposed person begins to understand that mastery of the potential health effects of the exposure will not be possible. In the process of attempting to be vigilant about an invisible exposure, the exposed person learns that the information necessary to make an informed adaptation to that exposure is simply not available. Instead of attaining a satisfactory means of maintaining vigilance over the consequences of the exposure, the exposed person encounters a fulminating wealth of experiential uncertainties and adaptational dilemmas.

In their attempts to gain mastery over this invisible threat, exposed persons who are concerned about an invisible exposure will attempt to maintain constant vigil over the effects of that exposure. They do this as a means of maximizing the possibility of finding the information that they need to protect themselves from that exposure. The atomic veteran carefully scrutinizes every symptom and change in his body to determine if it is a sign of incipient critical illness. The dairy farmer assiduously monitors his cattle's health and experiments endlessly to determine why his herd is sick. The Love Canal resident pursues every available governmental authority in efforts to persuade them to do the proper health studies—the studies that must be done if it is to ever be proven that the Love Canal is posing a health threat to the residents of the canal area. In this process vigilance becomes hypervigilance, which becomes, in and of itself, a time-consuming form of fixation to that exposure.

In consequence of this unsuccessful coping process, the cognitive conditions on which the exposee's original adaptation were based will change. At the outset, the exposed person believes that adequate time and information will be available for a successful adaptation to and mastery of that exposure. This is the fourth belief in Janis's tetrad of beliefs that mediate vigilance. However, as adaptation to a dangerous exposure is pursued, the adaptee's fourth belief changes to the assessment that mastery of the health effects of the exposure will not be possible.

With the change in this fourth belief, the conditions necessary for the pattern of hypervigilance come into existence. As we have already seen, hypervigilance is a predominant response to an invisible exposure. It is at this juncture that the belief in the danger of an invisible exposure becomes a fixation. Armed with the now-perceived difficulties of mastering the situation and with the simultaneous and paradoxical belief that successful adaptation to the exposure may still somehow be possible, the exposed person becomes hypervigilant. Hypervigilance develops as a means of maximizing the possibility of finding the information necessary for a successful adaptation. The implicit rationale of hypervigilance is that by maintaining constant vigil, an exposed person will ferret out and respond to any and all signs of the impending danger at the earliest possible juncture.

This approach to invisible threats seems understandable and may even have its strategic virtues. For example, it may actually generate the quickest possible response to a dangerous consequence of an invisible exposure. Nonetheless, this approach also takes a considerable psychic toll. Vigilance becomes hypervigilance as preoccupation with the contamination sets in. The exposed person's life becomes more and more focused on and limited to concerns about the endured contamination.

In addition, this sustained process of hypervigilance interacts with the process of creating a nonempirical belief system about an invisible exposure. Sustained hypervigilance helps to create the conditions that generate the development of nonempirical belief systems by people who have been exposed to an invisible contaminant. Vigilance based on the belief that an invisible exposure has been dangerous provides the exposed person with experience and evidence that stimulate the elaboration of this original belief into a larger belief system that portrays the dangers of that exposure.[47] For example, the discovery at Love Canal that many of the domestic animals that played near the canal developed rashes on their bellies[48] suggested to concerned neighborhood residents that the chemicals in the canal were causing these rashes. This conclusion strengthened the previous belief that these chemicals were also affecting the health of the human residents of the area. In a similar fashion, an atomic veteran's discovery that yet another of his former shipmates had been diagnosed as having a cancer makes him further convinced that he, too, has been harmed by radiation.

Thus the process of vigilance nurtures the growth of the nonempirical belief systems developed in response to an invisible exposure, and as a result these belief systems come to have a considerably larger scope of content than when they are first created. They grow to include more and more evidence about the exposure in question,[49] and they can begin to encompass altered beliefs about both the nature of society and the nature of the exposed person's own life.[50] As they grow, the nonempirical belief systems begin to provide exposed people with new images of self and world, which begin to supersede their prior images of self and world. The result is a dialectical or oscillatory relationship between the old and new imagery[51]—the same type of oscillation between old and new cognitive schema that Horowitz considers to be a characteristic symptom of the traumatic neuroses.[52] In addition, the new imagery of self and world embodied in a belief system developed in response to an invisible exposure can actually become a dominant mode of meaning for the exposed person. It gives cognitive support to the hypervigilant response to that exposure.

Thus it can be seen that the cognitive response to an invisible exposure strongly resembles the fixation process found in acute traumatic neuroses. Both involve the creation of and fixation to new images of world and self precipitated by a traumatic event. However, the cognitive response to these two types of trauma are different in two significant ways: (1) in the rapidity of onset of fixation and (2) in the content of the resultant fixation. Fixations developed in response to an acute and palpable trauma develop either immediately or within months. In the case of an invisible exposure, the fixation takes a much longer period of time to develop. In terms of content, in the instance of an acutely traumatic event, a fixation is developed that contains the imagery of the self and the world embodied in the traumatic event. However, in the case of an invisible exposure, the content of the fixation is different. The fixation embodies an imagery of the world and the self in which the exposed person has been contaminated and harmed by the exposure. With invisible exposure, the fixation does not directly reflect the original traumatic event. This new imagery is described by the nonempirical belief systems that the exposed persons develop in response to an invisible exposure. Over time exposed persons begin to live in this now-dangerous and contaminated world in much the same sense that the Vietnam veterans continue to live in the jungles of Vietnam.

In light of these considerations it is tempting to conclude that those people who have become cognitively and behaviorally fixated upon the consequences of an invisible exposure have developed a traumatic neurosis that is similar to the traumatic neuroses precipitated by an acute traumatic event. In both cases, the lack of mastery of a stressful event leads to a cognitive and behavioral fixation to that event. The only difference between the resultant neuroses, as we shall see, is their symptomatology.

Some evidence suggests that exposure to an invisible environmental contaminant actually causes development of a delayed-onset form of post-traumatic stress disorder. Three studies have demonstrated the occurrence of a traumatic neurosis in people who have been exposed to an invisible contaminant. Lifton found this phenomenon among Hiroshima survivors.[53] The entity that he found, called "A-Bomb Neurosis" by Hiroshima physicians, involved a preoccupation by survivors with the effects of radiation on their health. Brodsky found among his subjects a subgroup of patients who had developed traumatic neurosis in response to an occupational exposure to toxic chemicals.[54] I have described a syndrome developed by military veterans exposed to radiation that appears to be a delayed-onset form of post-traumatic stress disorder. This syndrome is described in chapter 14.

14
The Psychological Effects of Ionizing Radiation

This chapter is a case study of a group of military veterans who have developed an almost identical psychological response to their exposures to ionizing radiation. The similarity of both their experiences and their responses to those experiences is quite striking and can be described as a series of psychological symptoms that I call the radiation response syndrome (RRS).

Each of the subjects in this study was traumatized by his exposure to radiation. The veterans have been traumatized in the sense that they now live in realities that are both derivative of and defined by the traumatic experience of their exposure to radiation.

When this chapter was originally written (1982), I did not regard the radiation response syndrome as a form of posttraumatic stress disorder. I made this decision on the grounds that the symptoms of the syndrome were somewhat different than those of acute onset posttraumatic stress disorder. However, I have since changed my mind, and now regard the radiation response syndrome as a form of delayed onset posttraumatic stress disorder. I arrived at this conclusion on the basis of the similarity between the psychopathological processes involved in the development of both entities. My thinking on this matter is outlined in chapter 13. It seems possible that the symptoms of the RRS might, in fact, be the characteristic symptoms of a diagnostic entity called delayed-onset posttraumatic stress disorder. However, proof of the existence of this entity, as something different from chronic posttraumatic stress disorder, awaits further study. In addition, longitudinal population studies of the incidence, prevalence, and etiology of this diagnostic entity also remain to be done.

This is a case study of eleven atomic veterans. The atomic veterans are that group of men who actively participated, as members of the various branches of the U.S. military, in the atmospheric nuclear tests that this country con-

Reprinted with permission from *Culture, Medicine and Psychiatry* 7 (1983) 241–261. Copyright 1983 by *D. Reidel Publishing Company.*

ducted between the years of 1946 and 1962. This chapter will focus upon and describe the response of these men to the realization that they have been exposed to potentially dangerous doses of ionizing radiation. All of the subjects presented with a strikingly uniform complex of psychiatric symptoms. The symptoms appear to be a development upon the belief, held by each of these men, that they have been physically harmed by the radiation to which they were exposed. This self-diagnostic belief appears to have developed as a means of resolving the health mystery into which these men were placed by their exposure to ionizing radiation. Finally, these findings raise two additional questions: (1) is this symptom complex a pathogenetic development of a self-diagnostic belief into a larger set of psychiatric symptoms that elaborate upon and give expression to this belief? and (2) is the symptom complex a psychological consequence of exposure to nonbackground ionizing radiation?

It appears that somewhere in excess of 250,000 atomic veterans participated in atmospheric nuclear tests and that the nature of their participation varied. For example, many of them were placed in trenches one or two miles from the detonation site of a nuclear explosion. Twenty minutes after the explosion, these same men would march directly to ground zero for the purpose of executing routine military maneuvers. (This was the nature of subject number three's test participation.) Others, as crew on U.S. naval ships, steamed their way into ground zero hours after witnessing an explosion from the deck of a ship that had been positioned at a few miles of remove. (This was the nature of subject number seven's test participation.) Still others flew planes through newly formed mushroom clouds. The concept was to determine whether men and equipment were capable of functioning under post-detonation conditions.[1]

There have been innumerable reports indicating that ionizing radiation causes physiological disease.[2] However, reports indicating that radiation exposure can generate adverse psychological effects are rather scarce. The English literature contains only seven reports of adverse psychological effects in individuals exposed to nonbackground ionizing radiation. Such effects have been described in three populations: patients given therapeutic irradiation,[3] the survivors of Hiroshima, and the residents of the Three Mile Island area.[4] This chapter is a report on a fourth population group, and is the first description of a psychiatric symptom complex in individuals exposed to nonbackground ionizing radiation.

Method

In the fall of 1979 it was brought to our attention in the form of anecdotal reports that a significant number of atomic veterans were developing major psychological problems that they believed to be a consequence of their participation in atmospheric nuclear tests. A purposive sample of atomic

veterans was assembled to determine if there was any validity to this anecdotal hypothesis.

The sample was composed of members of the National Association of
Atomic Veterans (NAAV)—a fledgling advocacy group that had been formed
to address the individual and group problems of the atomic veterans. NAAV
had been developing a file of the names, military records, and chief medical
complaints of its members. It was from this file that the names of the subjects
were drawn. We asked NAAV to send us the names of those individuals who
met the following criteria: (1) they had complained of medical and/or psychological problems, and (2) they lived in California. In addition, it was also
established that none of the subjects had ever communicated with one
another prior to the time of the study.

We received approximately forty names from NAAV and interviewed the
first twelve men with whom appointments could be made. Potential subjects
were contacted, and permission to interview was requested. Each man who
agreed to participate was interviewed in depth. There were no refusals. Each
subject was interviewed on a number of occasions for a total period of time
varying from eight to fifteen hours.

Results

It seemed plausible that a group of men could be developing psychological
problems as a result of their participation in atmospheric nuclear tests. It was
thought that perhaps such an experience could deprive an individual of the
luxury of denying the realities of nuclear weapons, and that this psychological
predicament could, in turn, be producing the problems of which the atomic
veterans were complaining.

It turned out that this working hypothesis was not quite correct. Although some of the subjects were deeply concerned about nuclear weapons,
the most striking finding of this study has been that eleven of the first twelve
men we saw had developed an almost identical cluster of symptoms related to
their exposure to ionizing radiation. The similarity of these symptoms among
these men is striking and appears to comprise a syndrome. Before going on to
describe these symptoms, it will be helpful to first consider two additional
matters: (1) the typical posttest experience of the atomic veteran, and (2) the
mystery that the atomic veteran experiences as a result of this exposure to
ionizing radiation.

History of the Posttest Experience

The typical posttest atomic veteran experience has been characterized by
three phases: (1) the asymptomatic phase, (2) the symptomatic phase, and (3)
the syndrome phase.

The Asymptomatic Phase. The majority of the atomic veterans left the service believing that their health had not been impaired by the radiation to which they had been exposed. They held this belief because they had been taught, as part of their training or debriefing for the tests in which they participated, that they would not be harmed by the radiation. (There are exceptions to this trend. Three of the subjects of this study report that they were convinced at the time of their test participation that they had been harmed by exposure to radiation. However, all of these men claim to have forgotten their concerns until years later.)

During the asymptomatic phase, the atomic veterans were basically healthy and led relatively normal lives. Either they had no major illnesses, or they had routine illnesses that their physicians could readily diagnose and treat. This asymptomatic period varied in length from eight to eighteen years.

The Symptomatic Phase. The symptomatic phase was a period in which the eleven subjects developed physical illnesses that became central issues in their lives. Four of the subjects developed illnesses that could have been caused by ionizing radiation: leukemia, cataract, and basal cell carcinoma. Seven of them experienced a long series of major and minor physical illnesses that are not considered to be caused by ionizing radiation. All of them have developed a variety of physical symptoms that their physicians were unable to diagnose and/or treat. Some of these undiagnosable symptoms were genuinely debilitating and were the focus of extensive laboratory evaluation by their physicians.

Each of the subjects experienced unresolvable questions about their illnesses. The questions varied from man to man. The man with leukemia did not in his own mind understand why he had developed the leukemia. The men who were chronically ill could not understand why they were having so much difficulty with their health. The men with undiagnosable symptoms wanted diagnoses and treatment. Several subjects saw upwards of twenty physicians in their search for understanding, diagnosis, and treatment of their illnesses.

In the face of this experience, all eleven men continued to believe that radiation exposure had not harmed them. It was not until they were informed of the dangers of radiation (by either the mass media or the Department of Defense) that they began to consider the possibility that radiation could be causing their problems. This realization, in turn, appears to have triggered the onset of the syndrome phase.

The Syndrome Phase. The syndrome phase is characterized by the onset of the symptom complex mentioned earlier. The following case histories illustrate the manner in which these symptoms developed.

Case History No. 1

John is a forty-four-year-old white male who has been diagnosed as having dermatomyositis. He is a large man, who retains many marks of the professional athlete he once was. Underneath the bravado he is a man who is confused and hurt by the injustice he feels he has endured at the hands of his government. In his own words: "I'd be satisfied if they just said they were sorry." He hides his anger and pain behind a facade of humor.

John enlisted in the army at the age of seventeen and served in Korea. Afterwards he went to Nevada and participated in the Teapot series of nuclear tests. He installed and repaired communications lines, and he observed several tests from trenches.

After he left the service, he forgot about his test experiences. "The whole thing wasn't really all that important to me until 1972." In 1972 he became symptomatic. His symptoms included profound muscle weakness, arthralgias, and neuralgias. Once be became symptomatic, he was unable to work.

Before he received the diagnosis of dermatomyositis, he had seen eleven physicians in his attempt to find help for his medical problems. "I coulda jumped up and down and kissed the guy [diagnosing physician] when he told me what I had. I was beginning to wonder if I was crazy." Interestingly enough, some of the physicians who have seen John since his diagnosis do not concur with it. However, in John's mind, he has dermatomyositis.

John says that he has been through five stages with his illness:

At first I didn't believe that I was ill. Then I began to believe it, but eleven doctors told me I wasn't so I began to believe I was crazy. Then I found a doctor who could help me. After the excitement wore off, I found that every time I got a new symptom I'd pick up the phone and call my doctor, because I thought every new symptom meant I was going to die. Now, every time I get a new symptom, I give it a chance. I wait until the next morning to call the doctor.

At the present time, John spends most of his time at home alone or with his wife. He doesn't like to be around people anymore because "they expect me to be sociable." He spends most of his time at home working on or thinking about atomic veterans affairs. "For the last four years I've been obsessed with the atomic veteran stuff. It's a challenge. I'd like to win. I'd like to prove they were lying to us. We didn't know what we were doing. We were guinea pigs."

He is angry at the government and thinks "politicians" are to blame for the predicament he's in now. "What angers me most is that because of what the government did to me, all my loved ones suffer." He has found no relief from the Veterans Administration. "I think the VA tags us atomic veterans. We get tagged as psychological problems soon as they find out we're atomic veterans. You have to be on the defense when you go to the VA." John misses his old lifestyle dearly. "If there is something I'd love to do, it's bring home a paycheck."

Case History No. 2

Steve is a forty-nine-year-old male who is complaining of numerous physical ailments, the most prominent of which are neck pain of unknown etiology and recurrent gross hematuria of unknown etiology. He appears depressed and he has a difficult time smiling. He has the air of a worried man, and in fact he is constantly worrying about his health.

He served in the navy for four years. While doing a tour of duty on an aircraft carrier, he participated in a fifteen-megaton nuclear test—the Bravo shot. The shot scared him. "The average person just can't understand the power of a nuclear shot. It scares the hell out of you." The mushroom cloud from that test unexpectedly entered the jet stream and deposited gray radio-active ash on the carrier deck twenty minutes after detonation. The entire crew was ordered below deck immediately and stayed there for four days. He describes those four days as "scary," "muggy," and filled with a tension that erupted into frequent fights. "The uncertainty of not knowing what would happen was profound. We were all scared down to our socks."

The experience left its imprint on Steve's life. He says now that "ever since that test I've assumed that I was gonna die of cancer." At the same time, he claims that he never really thought about the danger of radiation until 1977, when he read a news story describing the details of another atomic veteran's fight with his illness and the Veterans Administration. The story reminded Steve of his own situation and convinced him that he was dying of an illness caused by radiation. "Until I read that story I thought I had a faint chance of escaping death at the hands of radiation." He says that he entered into an immediate and deep depression from which he has never recovered.

Steve is convinced that he is going to die soon and that radiation has caused the illness that will kill him. He feels that his mind and body are deteriorating, and he is, indeed, symptomatic. However, extensive medical evaluations have yet to yield a diagnosis. He has been told that he is a hypo-chondriac several times, but he does not believe it. He has, however, been humiliated by the process and has "started telling a shorter and shorter story each time I go to a new doctor—in hopes that they'll listen."

Steve is very angry about his present situation. He feels as though the government used him as a "guinea pig." He channels his anger into gathering information that will prove that radiation is harmful and that the government knew it at the time of the test. Any conversation with Steve is laced with facts and information that he feels will prove his point. In response to a question about how he can prove that the government knew that the tests were danger-ous for the atomic veterans, he answered as follows:

I think I can prove it. They took away my photographic gear before we left San Diego. They stationed the carrier fifty miles due east of ground zero and the prevailing wind there normally blows west. Finally, they rigged the ship to survive fallout. The hatches were resealed. An air re-breathing system was installed, and a system to automatically clean the outside of the boat was installed. They knew.

At the present time Steve is unemployed, although he had been consistently employed before 1977.

The syndrome that veterans develop during this third phase is characterized by four symptomatic processes: (1) a discomfort with the mystery surrounding exposure to ionizing radiation, (2) a preoccupation with the effects of ionizing radiation on health, (3) a series of identity conflicts precipitated by the changes that occurred in their lives subsequent to test participation, and (4) the development of a characteristic belief system about ionizing radiation. An understanding of these processes requires prior consideration of the mystery that accompanies exposure to ionizing radiation.

The Mystery

Once they were notified of the dangers of radiation, each of the subjects found himself getting submerged deeper and deeper in a compelling mystery concerning his physical health. This mystery was compelling in the sense that it demanded answers. Were my past illnesses caused by radiation? Will I develop a cancer? Why does my leg go numb? Will my children be normal?

The centerpiece of this mystery, but by no means its only facet, has been for most atomic veterans the undiagnosable somatic symptoms mentioned earlier. These symptoms, when present, truly alter the atomic veteran's existence.

There are, however, several other compelling elements to this mystery. They are generated by the following circumstances:

1. Ionizing radiation is an invisible contaminant. It is impossible to see, feel, or smell.

2. Once exposure to ionizing radiation has occurred, it is impossible for the exposed individual to determine if he has been injured until illness develops. This may take twenty to thirty years.

3. Once an individual becomes symptomatic from suspected radiation illness, it is almost impossible to prove that the illness has been caused by radiation. There is no clinical pathology of radiation lesions.

4. Once an individual becomes symptomatic from suspected radiation illness, it is impossible to know if and when that individual will develop additional illness.

The mystery is not, however, a complete one. It is a valenced mystery, in the sense that the exposed individual knows that ionizing radiation can definitely cause illness, but finds himself in the position of being unable to learn anything about the personal consequences of his own exposure.

The Atomic Veteran Response to the Mystery

Judging from the atomic veteran response to this situation, the mystery itself becomes problematic. All of the men in this series have made it clear that they are more than a little desperate about wanting to know how radiation has affected their health. Many of them have stated that they would even prefer to receive a fatal diagnosis than continue to receive no diagnosis at all. To quote one veteran, "To get a bad diagnosis is better than receiving no diagnosis at all. Otherwise you keep wondering about it."

In the face of this mystery, all of the subjects began to provide themselves with their own answers. They decided that they were ill and probably dying of an illness caused by ionizing radiation. All eleven believe that they have developed and are developing illnesses caused by radiation. Once an atomic veteran makes this decision, he goes on to develop a larger belief system about his exposure to ionizing radiation.

Each of the subjects of this study has independently developed a strikingly similar belief system about his exposure to ionizing radiation. This belief system is remarkable for its narrowness of scope and for the degree to which it dominates the manner in which the subjects see the world.

The major thematic consistencies found in the belief system of the atomic veteran are listed in chapter 11. Basically, the belief system holds that the men are dying, that doctors are of little help, that one doctor may exist who could help, that the government is to blame for their illness, and that people think they are crazy for blaming exposure to ionizing radiation for their illnesses.

As this belief system develops, it becomes a lens through which the atomic veteran sees the world. Eventually, he begins to act upon it. It is expressed in two symptomatic processes: (1) a preoccupation with his health and radiation, and (2) a series of identity conflicts.

The Preoccupation Dynamic

The preoccupation dynamic presents, in each veteran's behavior, as a virtual obsession with each of the following issues: (1) piecing together the circumstances of his own involvement in the nuclear tests, (2) proving that radiation caused his illness, (3) sometimes having to prove that he is really ill, (4) convincing the Veterans Administration and his family, friends, and greater society that all of the above are true, and (5) spending at least half of his waking time thinking and talking about these matters. This preoccupation can be quite debilitating. All of the men in this sample are chronically unemployed. This preoccupation also leads to social isolation. Friends and family drop away as the atomic veteran's preoccupation develops into a soliloquy. Usually the last person left is the veteran's wife. If she chooses to remain with him, she usually becomes enmeshed in her husband's concerns about radiation.

The veteran's preoccupation is involuntary, and is frequently experienced by the veteran as an intrusive and persistent stream of consciousness. The following dialogue with a man who has held forty-two jobs since he left the service illustrates this quality of preoccupation:

> —I can't pay attention and do things. My mind runs a lot during the day, and I have trouble going to sleep. Usually, I can't get to sleep until three in the morning.
>
> —*What is it that goes on in your mind?*
>
> —I think about ways to prove these problems.
>
> —*What do you mean by "prove these problems"?*
>
> —To prove that the radiation hurt me. And that the government lied. Then and now, I think a lot about what it will be like when we win our case. I have this fantasy in which I come in with the hard evidence and get $100,000 from the government. Then I get every last atomic veteran drunk and send my daughter to college.
>
> —*What else do you think about?*
>
> —I think an awful lot about giving my kids the things I'd give them if I were able to hold a job. I'd buy them a pool and take them on trips. I'd buy track shoes for my son.

This preoccupation also intrudes into the dreams of atomic veterans. The following dialogue occurred with a man who had been in a trench that he estimated to have been a mile and a half from ground zero of an explosion.

> —Fifty percent or more of my waking time is spent thinking about the explosion. It has been that way since 1978.
>
> —*What triggered it?*
>
> —The first dream—which was about the trench. I was scared, sweating and screaming. Other men were screaming too. Have you ever heard a grown man cry? The dreams occur once or twice a week now. After the dreams, I don't feel like eating, *It's like being there.*
>
> —*Why do you think you keep reliving it?*
>
> —I don't know.

Identity Conflict

The identity conflict dynamic is a consequence of the identity changes that have occurred in the adult life of the atomic veterans subsequent to their exposure to ionizing radiation. Each of the men in this series sees himself as being a different person as a result of his exposure to ionizing radiation. Three perceived transitions have consistently occurred in the lives of these atomic veterans: (1) the transition from being healthy to being unhealthy, (2) the transition from perceiving one's self as patriotic to perceiving one's self as being unpatriotic, and (3) the transition from being a connected social individual to being an isolated, asocial individual. Conflicts between the veteran's old and new identity ensue, and they surface as the defenses that the veterans developed to avoid admitting that these changes had, in fact, occurred.

This dynamic was first observed in an interview with an atomic veteran who is partially blind now as a result of bilateral cataracts and several retinal detachments. During an extended discussion about the seeming contradiction between being angry at one's government and being patriotic, this man discovered that he had resolved this conflict by deciding that it was unpatriotic to question his government's actions. This conflict had even affected his perception of his own illness:

—It has been hard for me to admit that radiation caused my cataracts.
—*Why?*
—Because that means that the government caused them.
—*Why is that a problem?*
—Because I'm a loyal American and it screws up my mind to be at odds with the government. I'd serve again tomorrow, if I had to, but not at Eniwetok.

Similar defenses developed in response to other identity transitions. Many veterans have had a profound resistance to admitting that they are irreversibly ill. For example, one man who has been diagnosed as having a crippling muscular disease still cherishes the belief that he will one day return to his prior work as a professional athlete.

Atomic veterans have also had difficulty accepting the transition to social isolation. Resistance to isolation appears as a variety of defenses. Most atomic veterans have decided that other people think they are crazy, and almost all of them insist that only people who have experienced a nuclear explosion can understand the atomic veteran.

The following dialogue is illustrative:

—I'm down to two friends; most people think I'm crazy. They say it's a disgrace to say what I say.
—*Why?*
—Because they think it's important for our country to be strong—like a strong man who can fight his way out of any situation. But you can be strong in your mind instead.

—*How do you feel about being called crazy?*

—I'm willing to be called crazy. I'm gonna go for it. I'd rather be alone anyway. That way I don't have to argue with them. They don't know what
they're talking about. I was there. I do.

Discussion

The Radiation Response Syndrome

All eleven atomic veterans studied here have developed a virtually identical
complex of psychiatric symptoms. The complex appears to be a syndrome.
This syndrome—which we are calling, for the sake of present discussion, the
radiation response syndrome—has two basic components: (1) an elaborate
belief system centered around a core belief that one has been physically harmed
by ionizing radiation, and (2) a set of behavioral symptoms that appear to be
a direct expression of the contents of this belief system.

The RRS, as it presented in the subjects of this series, is a debilitating
condition. It is not a simple fear of radiation. The syndrome is debilitating in
two senses: (1) it has disrupted the social fabric of the lives of these men.
Their ability to maintain normal social relationships with their family and
friends has been severely compromised by the preoccupation component of
the syndrome. (2) It has become impossible for these men to hold onto their
jobs. At the present time, none of the subjects is employed. They were all
regularly employed for long periods of time after their participation in nuclear
tests.

Differential Diagnosis

The RRS bears a resemblance to posttraumatic stress disorder (PTSD), somatization disorder, and hypochondriacal neurosis. It appears to be similar to
PTSD in that a single stressor or event (participation in an atmospheric
nuclear test) may have been the cause of a major change in the lives of these
men. However, the subjects are not really preoccupied with a past event in
the same sense that one is in PTSD. The atomic veterans do not generally
reexperience the tests in which they participated, although this does occasionally occur. They are, instead, preoccupied with radiation and its impact
on their lives. In addition, the time of onset of RRS is different from that of
PTSD. Symptoms of the RRS did not develop until more than a decade after
test involvement.

The picture of somatization disorder is similar to the picture of the RRS,
in that both entities present with multiple somatic complaints that appear
to be functional. They differ in their age of onset (less than twenty-five years

of age for somatization disorder), and in the fact that almost all of the atomic veterans in this study had developed documented organic disease as well as seemingly functional illnesses.

The picture of hypochondriasis bears considerable resemblance to the preoccupation component of the RRS. The hypochondriacal patient is "dominated by *preoccupation* with the body and with fear of presumed disease of various organs."[5] Nemiah describes the hypochondriacal person as a patient who "presents his complaints at length, in detail, and with an urgent insistent pressure of speech that rarely allows the physician to get a word in edgewise."[6] The same could be said of the subjects in this series.

Despite these similarities, there appear to be some important differences between these two groups of patients. The hypochondriacal patient presents with purely functional symptoms. This is not the case with the atomic veterans. As shown in table 14–1, nine of the subjects developed documented organic disease well before they had ever developed the symptoms of the RRS.

In a similar vein, the course of events leading up to development of the RRS suggests that the RRS and hypochondriacal neurosis involve two different psychological processes. In contrast to the hypochondriac, who appears to be a person in search of an illness, *the atomic veteran is a person in search of meaning for a disease that he has already developed.* Consider the following developmental sequence of events, which was identical for all of the subjects in this study.

1. The veterans returned home from their participation in nuclear tests with the firm belief that they were healthy and unendangered by the radiation to which they had been exposed.

2. After differing periods of time (almost always more than ten years after test involvement) they developed somatic problems that posed, for each of them, at least one unanswerable medical question.

3. Eventually, they were notified (either by the Department of Defense, the mass media, or a physician) that the radiation to which they were exposed might have been dangerous.

4. They decided that their illness was related to ionizing radiation.

5. They developed the symptoms of the RRS.

In other words, the atomic veterans were men who had been unable, prior to notification, to give meaning to the various somatic illnesses that they were experiencing. They were unable to give meaning to their illnesses because they could not obtain answers to a number of central questions about those illnesses.

7	Deceased	Navy	2	Bikini: Operation Crossroads. Located on ship 10 miles from GZ. Then lived on ship that had been in target area at time of test (22 days).	1. COPD 2. Cataracts 3. Bursitis
8	51	Navy	1	Bikini: Teak shot. Observed test from deck of ship at distance of 150 miles. Ship returned to GZ within 6 hours	1. Diverticulosis 2. Hypertension 3. Calcified granulomas of lung 4. Various skin lesions
9	47	Army	6	Nevada Test Site: Operation Teapot. Positioned in trenches 2500 yards from GZ. Marched down to GZ three times.	1. Dermatomyositis 2. Basal Cell Carcinoma ($\times 3$)
10	47	Marines	2	Nevada Test Site. Positioned in trenches 2 miles from GZ. Walked down to GZ.	1. Neuromuscular symptoms of unknown etiology
11	49	Air Force	1	Bravo Shot. Stationed on island 125 miles from GZ. Fallout fell on island because of windshift.	1. Encephalitis 2. Hiatal hernia 3. Child with Down's Syndrome 4. Recurrent nosebleeds.

[a] As reported by subject.
[b] GZ = ground zero.
[c] Chronic Obstructive Pulmonary Disorder.

It is a set of beliefs and ideas in which a person decides that he has a disease caused by ionizing radiation. As such, it would appear to be a variety of belief system concerned with etiology.

This belief system has a two-part structure: (1) a central self-diagnostic belief (SDB) that one's body has been harmed by ionizing radiation and (2) a set of ancillary beliefs that elaborate upon and give support to the self-diagnostic belief. The ancillary beliefs seem to fall into two basic categories: expressive beliefs and dialectical beliefs.

Expressive beliefs are, more or less, ideas that develop or extend the SDB. An example might be the belief that one's children will have birth defects; or the statement that "138 of the guys on my boat have developed cancer."

Dialectical beliefs are ideas generated in response to people and situations that have disagreed with or challenged the veteran's SDB. An example might be the belief that the Veterans Administration is not giving compensation and medical care to the atomic veterans because it is trying to cover up the fact that radiation is dangerous; or the belief that doctors don't know anything about radiation. In and of themselves, these beliefs are not pathological. They appear to be pathological only to the extent that they are part of the RRS.

All of the component ideas of this SDBS can be understood as inferences upon the SDB. Consider, as one example, the atomic veteran's attitude toward his physicians. Because he believes that he has a disease caused by radiation, he regards the physician who tells him otherwise as dishonest.

A similar relationship appears to exist between the self-diagnostic belief system and the behavioral symptoms of the RRS. These symptoms appear to be a behavioral elaboration and expression of this belief system. They are the behavior of a person who believes that he has been physically injured by ionizing radiation. Consider the following examples:

1. Because he believes that he has a physical radiation injury, the atomic veteran tends to look at every change in the status of his body as the first sign of the cancer that he *knows* he is going to develop. The cut that takes too long to heal sets him to wondering if he has leukemia. The headache that persists for three days suggests a brain tumor. The weakness in his left arm could be anything. He becomes preoccupied with his health, and with understanding how radiation has affected it.

2. Because he is preoccupied with his health and radiation, he becomes a different man in his own eyes and the eyes of his family and friends. He stops talking about his old interests and spends most of his time thinking and talking about radiation-related matters. His relationships deteriorate under the strain of his preoccupation.

3. Because he believes that he has a radiation injury, the atomic veteran looks at the government agency that tells him he is incorrect as dishonest and irresponsible. At the same time, he believes that he is being unpatriotic for holding such an opinion.

In other words, not only do these men believe that they have been harmed by radiation; they also think and behave as though they have been. The question remains as to whether or not the belief actually causes the behavior to develop.

Pathogenetic Hypothesis

From the foregoing analysis, we know that three generalizations can be made about the radiation response syndrome as it presented among the subjects of this study:

1. The symptoms of the syndrome developed after the atomic veterans decided that they had been harmed by ionizing radiation.
2. The self-diagnostic belief system contained in the radiation response syndrome appears to be a group of inferences upon the self-diagnostic belief.
3. The behavioral symptoms of the radiation response syndrome appear to be both congruent with and an exact expression of the self-diagnostic belief system and the conflicts that it precipitates.

Taken together, these generalizations suggest the following hypothesis about the pathogenesis of the RRS: The radiation response syndrome is a pathological development of the self-diagnostic belief (that one has been physically injured by radiation) into the symptoms that are the radiation response syndrome. This hypothesis is testable, and is being assessed in our own prospective population studies at Three Mile Island as discussed below.

Etiology

Radiation. It is, of course, impossible to determine the etiology of the RRS from the present series. This is a case study, and in the nature of case studies, the sample is small and has not been randomly selected. Proper assessment of the prevalence, etiology, and pathogenesis of the RRS will require controlled population studies of the atomic veterans and other populations exposed to nonbackground ionizing radiation (NBIR)

Nonetheless, the findings of the present study raise the question of whether or not development of the RRS is somehow related to or caused by exposure to NBIR. The symptomatic content of the syndrome is primarily concerned with ionizing radiation, and all of the men in this series were exposed to NBIR as participants in atmospheric nuclear tests.

Two types of studies lend support to the hypothesis that development of the RRS is related to radiation exposure. Lifton's study of Hiroshima survivors actually demonstrated the presence of RRS-like symptoms in this population. One of his many findings at Hiroshima was that a number of the survivors developed "a lifelong preoccupation with [leukemia]—with blood counts and bodily complaints, particularly that of weakness—to the extent of greatly restricting their lives or even becoming bedridden."[9] These symptoms were common in Hiroshima. In contrasting the symptoms of this "neurosis" to other entities, Lifton says that "as compared to usual hypochondriacal and phobic patterns encountered in psychiatric work, those in [A-bomb neurosis] are much more directly related to actual bodily assaults that can result from atomic bomb exposure.[10] Once again, we see a hypochondriaform pattern in people exposed to NBIR.

The second type of study that suggests an etiological relationship between exposure and the RRS are a group of studies that have been done at Three Mile Island.[11] These studies have demonstrated that a large portion of the TMI area population has already developed the SDB and related beliefs. The most direct assessment of this phenomenon is found in a survey done by the Field Research Corporation in September of 1980. This survey (N = 2,033) found that 22 percent of the population living within five miles of TMI had already developed the belief that they had received "a dangerous dose of radiation during the accident." The same survey found that 50 percent of the population living within 25 miles of TMI believed that they would get a dangerous dose of radiation in the future.[12]

These studies also suggest that in and of itself, exposure to NBIR is not sufficient cause for development of an SDB or the RRS. For example, the Field survey also demonstrates that 78 percent of their sample did not develop an SDB.[13] In addition everyday clinical experience suggests that the vast majority of people receiving diagnostic medical x-rays never develop the RRS or an SDB. Clearly, factors other than the fact of radiation exposure must play a role in the development of the RRS.

It appears that one of these factors is the circumstances in which exposure occurs. For example, it is rare indeed to find someone who is concerned about the health effects of the background radiation to which we are all being constantly exposed. On the other hand, the existence of SDBs has been documented in three populations: Hiroshima survivors,[14] atomic veterans, and the residents of the Three Mile Island area.[15]

The present study suggests that yet another factor is the exposed individual's health status subsequent to radiation exposure. All of the subjects of this study developed either actual or perceived illnesses of significant proportion subsequent to their exposure to radiation. These illnesses seem to have convinced each of the subjects that they had been harmed by the radiation to which they had been exposed. These illnesses had first been a source of medical mystery for each of the subjects; they resolved this mystery by deciding that their illnesses were caused by ionizing radiation.

The consistency of this last set of findings suggests a hypothesis to explain the origins of the SDB: The self diagnostic belief that one has been physically harmed by ionizing radiation develops as a means of resolving any one of the various medical mysteries that an individual can experience subsequent to exposure to non-background ionizing radiation. Exposure to non-background ionizing radiation generates and permits development of a medical mystery because it is almost always empirically impossible to ascertain if an individual has been physically injured by a radiation exposure.

Thus it seems probable that *if* radiation exposure plays a role in causing development of the RRS, it does so because it has the potential to immerse an individual in a compelling medical mystery. If this is the case, then it also seems possible that an RRS-like syndrome is not specific to radiation exposure. It seems at least theoretically possible that this type of symptomatology could occur in response to any exposure that has the potential to immerse the exposed individual in a medical mystery.

Factors Unrelated to Radiation. It also seems possible that factors unrelated to radiation exposure may play a major role in the development of the RRS. Two types of variables should be systematically investigated: (1) the role of personality structure in the development of the RRS and (2) the role of perceived secondary gains in the development of the RRS.

In investigating the role of personality structure in the development of the RRS, two possibilities should be considered: (1) that individuals with a certain type of personality structure are more apt to develop the RRS and (2) that the RRS is actually the response of a specific type of character disorder to exposure to ionizing radiation. Nothing in the present study suggests that this is the case, but thorough psychiatric evaluation of a large random sample of atomic veterans is necessary to properly assess these possibilities.

In considering the possible role of secondary gain in the development of the RRS, two motives should be considered: (1) that the subjects of this study made the decision that they had been harmed by radiation in order to secure financial compensation and (2) that this decision was made as a means of escaping from a dysfunctional life by assuming a sick role. Once again, the present study does not suggest that either of these motives played a significant role in the development of the RRS; proper assessment of these possibilities will require psychiatric evaluation of a large random sample of atomic veterans.

Finally, it seems possible that the RRS is simply the response of an individual seeking retribution for a perceived injustice; the perceived injustice being, in this case, that the federal government is not compensating the subjects for injuries they believe they received in the military service. Our findings indicate that the factor of perceived injustice does play a role in shaping the *content* of the symptoms of the RRS. It does not, however, appear to be the cause of the syndrome. We have interviewed a considerable number of atomic veterans who have not developed the RRS but have developed a considerable amount of anger at the federal government because of what they perceive to be an injustice.

Conclusions and Future Research

This chapter presents a series of eleven atomic veterans who have developed an almost identical complex of psychiatric symptoms. The symptoms appear to comprise a syndrome. The development of these symptoms appears to be related to the subject's exposure to nonbackground ionizing radiation.

Specifically, the findings of this study suggest three hypotheses:

1. The radiation response syndrome is a pathological development of the self-diagnostic belief (that one has been physically harmed by ionizing radiation) into a set of symptoms that elaborate upon and express the self-diagnostic belief.
2. The self-diagnostic belief develops as a means of resolving any one of the various medical mysteries that an individual can experience subsequent to exposure to NBIR.
3. Development of the RRS is a consequence of exposure to NBIR.

These hypotheses can be tested by three types of research:

1. Additional clinical research on other groups of individuals exposed to NBIR,
2. Retrospective population studies of the atomic veterans, and
3. Prospective population studies of individuals recently exposed to NBIR (for example, the TMI area population).

It seems important to pursue further study of these phenomena because the findings of the present study raise the question of whether or not exposure to NBIR can cause, as a general phenomenon, adverse psychological effects.

15
Interlude

Modern stress research began with the work of Hans Selye at McGill University. Selye studied the physiological response of the mammalian body to physiological, as opposed to psychological, stressors. He found that the mammalian body responds to stressors in a nonspecific fashion; that is, it mounts a nearly identical physiological response to each of the different physiological stressors. The purpose of this nonspecific response is to protect an organism from the threats posed to its health by the stressors in question. Selye gave the name of general adaptation syndrome to this protective response of the body.

Selye found that in addition to protecting an organism from external threat, the general adaptation syndrome can also do damage to the mammalian body in which that reaction takes place. The general adaptation syndrome can also cause tissue damage and the development of a variety of diseases. Selye gave the name *diseases of adaptation* to the illnesses caused by the operation of the general adaptation syndrome. The central idea in this conception is that in its efforts to adapt to and protect itself from external stressors, the body does damage to itself. Selye considers peptic ulcers, hypertension, and myocardial infarcts to be examples of diseases of adaptation.[1]

In the same sense that the process of adaptation can cause somatic diseases of adaptation, adaptation to psychological stressors can also cause psychological diseases of adaptation. "Chronic stress is associated with psychiatric problems, negative emotional states, depression, anxiety and psychosomatic illness [of all kinds]."[2] In studying the psychological effects of an invisible contamination, it appears that we have discovered yet another instance of the harmful effects of an adaptive process.

In summary, we have gathered evidence that suggests that there are five types of untoward psychological consequences of attempting to adapt to an invisible exposure. The method that we have used has been one of looking at the existing case studies and finding that each of these different effects has occurred in a variety of circumstances involving exposure to the invisible contaminants. The five untoward effects that we have found by using this method are as follows:

1. Experienced uncertainty
2. Adaptive dilemmas
3. Nonempirical belief systems in which the exposed person portrays himself or herself as either being injured by an invisible exposure or as living or working in a situation in which invisible contaminants are a threat to health
4. Hypervigilance
5. Traumatic neuroses.

Our findings also suggest that each of these effects arises in consequence of attempting to adapt to an invisible exposure.

Successful adaptation to a psychological stressor or a threatening situation involves: (1) gathering information that permits effective adaptation to that threat and (2) mastering the threatening situation by responding to it in the manner suggested by the acquired information. Adaptation to an exposure to one or more of the invisible environmental contaminants will always be hindered by the fact that the information needed to successfully adapt to that exposure is not available. Because the invisibility of these contaminants renders it almost impossible to obtain the needed information, people exposed to and concerned with adapting to an invisible environmental contaminant find themselves trapped in a chronic state of encounter with a threat to their health that they cannot master.

At the same time that it is possible to begin to describe and define the adverse psychological effects of the invisible exposures, we really cannot say that we understand very much about these adverse effects. Even though we know something about the mechanisms by which they are brought into being, there is much that remains unknown. For example, we do not know why some people become hypervigilant in response to an invisible exposure and others do not. We know that most of the people who become hypervigilant are exposees who have had health problems subsequent to an invisible exposure. Yet not everyone who has health problems becomes hypervigilant. So health problems subsequent to an exposure will not necessarily produce exposee hypervigilance. In addition, we know that some people become hypervigilant even if they do not have problems with their health as a result of an exposure. For some people, exposure alone will set off a sequence of events that will lead them to hypervigilance. Carroll Brodsky[3] has described two groups of workers with illness careers. One of these groups was characterized by the presence of hypervigilant behavior prior to the appearance of their somatoform symptoms. Thus one is forced to conclude that not only does illness subsequent to an invisible exposure not invariably generate hypervigilance, but hypervigilance frequently develops in the absence of such illness.

The list of unanswered questions about hypervigilance is longer than this. All we really know is that it can occur in consequence of an invisible contamination. The same may be said of our knowledge of all of the other adverse psychological effects of the invisible exposures. We do not know why some people are deeply traumatized by an invisible exposure while others are not. We do not know why some people construct belief systems that portray an exposure as dangerous while others portray the same exposure as being safe.

Another interesting and unanswered basic question is a quantitative one. The question is this: In a given group of people exposed to an invisible contaminant, what percentage of those people will become vigilant about that exposure? This question comes from the recognition that some people will be concerned about an invisible exposure while others will simply not think about it at all. I suspect that a series of population studies of both exposed and unexposed populations would find that a fairly constant proportion of any population both will and will not be concerned with adapting to an invisible exposure. Such figures would give us some ideas as to how many people would generally be at risk, in an exposed population, of developing the adverse psychological effects of an invisible exposure. Such studies might also permit one to study the constitutional and situational differences that account for this difference in response to an exposure.

Another set of unanswered questions regards the relationship between the various psychological effects of an invisible exposure: Is hypervigilance a preliminary stage on the way to developing the radiation response syndrome? Does a comparable syndrome develop in people who have been exposed to the toxic chemicals? What proportion of hypervigilant people go on to develop the full gamut of syndrome symptoms? What is the relationship between hypervigilance and the development of belief systems?

Yet another set of unanswered questions regards the psychological consequences of public policy. It appears, as we shall see in the following chapters, that public policy can have major effects on the psychological response of an exposed population to an invisible contamination. The Department of Defense and the Veterans Administration, by electing not to help the atomic veterans cope, in a systematic fashion, with the health effects of the tests in which they participated, created conditions that encouraged those men to become preoccupied with their health. In a similar fashion, the state government of New York, in deciding to tell ring III residents that their Love Canal neighborhood was safe, only postponed the necessary decision of evacuating them from that area, and generated a significant amount of alienation, anger, uncertainty, and hypervigilance in that community. As these examples suggest, there is much to be learned about making the policy decisions in situations involving an invisible contamination.

Returning to what we do know, we can state that the central psychological fact of an invisible exposure is the experience of uncertainty. Many individuals who have been exposed to an invisible contaminant and who are concerned with protecting themselves from that exposure will be conspicuously burdened with and often consumed by the uncertainties that they experience as a result of trying to adapt to that exposure. This is a dramatic preoccupation that is evident to anyone who has had the opportunity to spend time with such a person.

The uncertainty feeds upon itself, and it becomes the breeding ground for the remaining psychological effects of the invisible contaminants. The cognitive, or experienced, uncertainty becomes in turn the source of the remaining psychological effects of an invisible exposure. This sequence of events can be portrayed as shown in figure 15–1. The diagram illustrates that attempts to adapt to an invisible exposure are usually precipitated by either the exposure itself or by the development of health problems subsequent to an exposure. In turn, attempts at adaptation generate uncertainty and adaptational failures. These conditions become the cognitive ground from which the remaining adverse psychological effects of the invisible environmental contaminants develop.

Uncertainty gives rise to adaptation dilemmas because the exposed person is unable to obtain the information he or she needs to adapt successfully to the threats posed by that exposure. Uncertainty gives rise to nonempirical belief systems because adaptation must go on anyway in the absence of adequate empirical information about a threat. As a result, exposed persons construct appraisals of an invisible threat as a means of providing themselves with some kind of cognitive ground on which they can mount an adaptation.

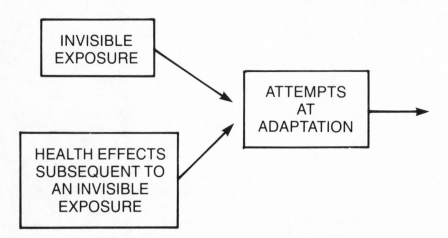

Figure 15–1. The Psychological Effects of the Invisible Environmental Contaminants

Uncertainty can also give rise to hypervigilance. It does so because it creates the cognitive conditions that give rise to hypervigilance: the simultaneous and paradoxical belief that successful adaptation to a serious threat is in theory possible, but because of circumstances not within reach. Finally, it appears that the traumatic neuroses may simply be a convergence and intensification of the previously mentioned psychological effects of an invisible exposure.

The adverse psychological effects of an invisible exposure, as listed above, are traumatic only when they are part of a fixation and/or preoccupation process. This means that with the exception of the traumatic neuroses, each of the above psychological effects may or may not be of a traumatic nature. A nonempirical belief system developed in response to an invisible exposure may be part of a process by which an exposed person becomes fixated on that exposure, or it may simply be a nonempirical appraisal of an invisible threat. In the same vein, hypervigilant behavior may be a temporary affair or it may be part of a persistent, and thus traumatic, response to an invisible exposure.

The following chapters consider the conditions that play a role in exacerbating the psychological effects of the invisible contaminants. All of these conditions exacerbate the traumatogenic dynamic because they increase the exposed person's sense of uncertainty about the consequences of the exposure in question. A common denominator present in each of the traumatogenic conditions is as follows: these conditions are situations in which the exposed people are given an inaccurate portrayal of the health effects of their exposures by either an individual or institution. For example, the Veterans

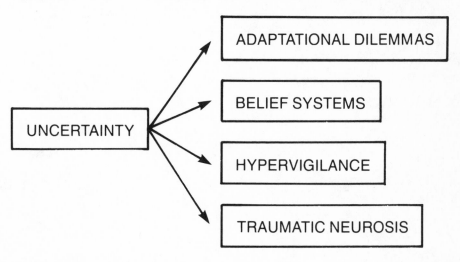

Administration might tell an atomic veteran that his lymphoma has not been caused by radiation even though the state of knowledge about the causes of his lymphoma must be characterized as one of etiological uncertainty. The uranium mining industry might not inform its miners of their increased risk of lung cancer, even though there is well-established scientific evidence that a substantial risk exists.

The psychological consequences of this type of behavior for exposed persons is an increase in their experienced uncertainty. Their uncertainty increases because an inaccurate portrayal of an invisible threat confuses their knowledge and appraisal of that threat, which makes adaptation to the threat more difficult. Three exacerbating dilemmas will be considered in the remaining portion of this book: (1) dysfunctional medical relationships, (2) blaming the victim, and (3) institutional denial of invisible threat.

16
Dysfunctional
Medical Relationships

The paucity of information concerning an invisible enviromental contamination leaves the exposed person feeling totally unable to monitor the health effects of the contaminant to which he or she was exposed. This same information deficit also disrupts a physician's ability to perform the normal functions of the doctor-patient relationship for the exposed patient. The medical relationship between the exposed patient and his or her physician becomes the primary arena in which the exposed person learns that successful empirical adaptation to a received invisible exposure will not be possible. The doctor-patient relationship is the place where the exposed person learns, in one fashion or another, that he or she will not be able to maintain effective vigilance over the health effects of a previous invisible exposure.

It is in the process of turning to a physician for help that the exposed person learns that no one, including the physicians, will be able to adduce the information necessary to appraise the health effects of an invisible exposure. As a result, the relationship that develops between the person who has been exposed to an invisible contaminant and his or her physicians often becomes dysfunctional and discordant. In this setting, patient vigilance will be transformed into hypervigilance, in response to the adaptational dilemmas and uncertainties that are generated by the medical invisibility of the invisible contaminants.

Physicians do not generally regard this hypervigilance as a hypertrophied form of a patient's normal needs for vigilance over his or her health. Instead they see this hypervigilance as a form of hypochondriasis. The result is an unfortunate and unnecessary vicious (positive feedback) cycle in which the exposed person is simultaneously blamed for (1) the medical invisibility of the illnesses caused by an invisible contaminant and (2) his or her wish to maintain vigilance over the possible health effects of the exposure to an invisible contaminant. As a result, the doctor-patient relationship becomes the source of considerable frustration and discomfort for the patient. For these reasons I have chosen to characterize those unfulfilling relationships that sometimes develop between the exposed patient and his or her physicians as dysfunctional medical relationships.

Before discussing in detail the topography of this medical dysfunction, we should first discuss the nature of the vigilance needs that the person exposed to an invisible contaminant brings to his or her physician's office.

Perhaps the first thing to be said about the person who is concerned about the health effects of an invisible exposure is that the exposure dramatically changes the nature of that person's relationship to his or her body. Most of us regard ourselves as having healthy bodies and carry around a minimal amount of concern about the various changes that routinely occur in our bodily states. However, many of the people who have been exposed to an invisible contaminant regard their bodies in a different fashion: They believe that their bodies have been or may have been damaged because they are contaminated. This perception of their bodies comprises a sort of middle state between being ill and being healthy.

Lifton, for example, found this phenomenon among the survivors of the bombing of Hiroshima. He described it as a survivor belief that an "enduring taint" has become attached to their bodies and lives.[1] I found in the case study presented in chapter 14 that the atomic veterans developed a self-diagnostic belief that they had been physically injured by the radiation to which they had been exposed.[2] Brodsky found similar beliefs among workers occupationally exposed to toxic chemicals.[3]

At this point only limited data are available to indicate how extensive this perception of bodily damage or contamination is, in an exposed population, but some studies do begin to bear upon this question. For example, at Three Mile Island, where a relatively small amount of radiation was released compared to Hiroshima or Chernobyl, there is some indication that a rather sizable portion of the TMI area population came to regard itself as contaminated or potentially contaminated by ionizing radiation. The prevalence of this attitude was most directly measured by a public opinion poll taken by Field Research Corporation in the Three Mile Island area fifteen months after the accident.[4] The poll showed that of people living within five miles of the plant, 14 percent believed that they got a dangerous dose of radiation, 60 percent believed they did not, and 25 percent didn't know. Almost half of these people believed they stood a chance of getting a dangerous dose of radiation in the future. Of those living five to twenty-five miles from the plant, only 8 percent believed they had gotten a dangerous dose of radiation, while 72 percent believed they had not. However, 41 percent believed they stood a chance of getting a dangerous dose in the future.

A study by Houts et al.[5] showed that of those people living within five miles of the TMI plant, 54 percent believed cancer rates would probably or definitely increase because of the accident. Of those living forty-one to fifty-five miles from the plant, 56 percent agreed. My survey[6] of the TMI area population showed that of people living within five miles of the plant, 24 percent strongly believed that they or someone they know would eventually get cancer because of the accident. These figures indicate: (1) that within fifteen months of the accident, 14 percent of the 40,000 people living within five miles of Three Mile Island, or 5,600 people, believed that they had been contaminated by the accident and (2) that approximately half of this same population still felt, two and three years later, that the radiation released by the accident presented them with a palpable and future threat to their health. These studies only begin to assess the extent to which an exposed population will regard itself as contaminated, but they are all that we have at this time.

Quantitative considerations aside, we can see that many of the people exposed to an invisible contaminant will come to regard their bodies as being actually or potentially contaminated by the exposure. The person who believes that his or her body has been or might have been contaminated by an invisible exposure will understandably want to monitor his or her health carefully, as a means of insuring the early detection and treatment of any contaminant-caused illness that might appear. As a result, these people become concerned with and sensitive to all of the changes that occur in their bodies.

The people who become most convinced of the contaminated status of their bodies and thus most concerned with being vigilant about potential contaminant-caused illness are those who develop significant health problems subsequent to an invisible exposure. The development of significant post-exposure illness seems to suggest to the exposed person that he or she has been or may have been physically injured by the invisible contaminant to which they were exposed. Consider, for example, the case of an atomic veteran named Oliver.[7] Oliver was stationed at Eniwetok Atoll in the South Pacific during a time in which six nuclear weapons tests were exploded there. He remembers "the good times at Eniwetok very well," and he says that "you couldn't explain the destructive power [of the bombs] to anyone. They'd never believe you." He also says that after leaving Eniwetok, "that power was the only [part of the experience that] I thought about until I learned [in 1977] about radiation damage. I'll probably be concerned about radiation effects for a long time to come."

Since his participation in the weapons testing program, Oliver has had a number of problems with his health. They are as follows:

1. Multiple skin cancers on his face.
2. Bilateral increased intraocular pressure of unknown etiology. (Increased intraocular pressure is the cardinal symptom of glaucoma, but Oliver's physicians have determined that his condition is not glaucoma.)
3. Transient Bell's Palsy of unknown etiology. (Bell's Palsy is a hemilateral paralysis of the facial muscles.)

4. Undiagnosed muscle symptoms of unknown etiology that include decreased muscle tone, exertional muscle pain and swelling, and decreased muscle strength.

5. Profound fatigue: "I feel like half a person. I have almost no mobility or energy."

6. Tinnitus: a constant ringing sensation in his right ear.

In addition, Oliver has also had one daughter who was born with four kidneys and "who was a very sick girl for most of her twenty years." All of Oliver's health problems became clinically apparent before he became aware that radiation could have harmed him, and he says that he never thought about the possibility until he watched a television program about radiation in 1977.

Oliver now says that ever since he learned that the radiation to which he was exposed might have harmed him, "I think I spend a lot of time thinking about my symptoms. When a new symptom appears, I wonder how bad it could be. I keep an eye on it. I watch it. If anything develops I'll be right down at the Veterans Administration." He says that he pays a lot of attention to his symptoms because he thinks it will help his doctors figure out what is going on.

Oliver is actually scared of his health and body, and of the effects that radiation may have had upon him: "It puts me in a life of fear. The fear that some of the symptoms I have now can turn into more serious disease. I've been very concerned about my eyesight. Given that they can't even say I have glaucoma, I don't really know what will happen. To get a bad diagnosis would be better than no diagnosis, because you keep wondering about it."

Oliver's response to radiation exposure is by no means unique. Another veteran, Ronald, describes himself as having been the kind of person who never had a doctor. "But now," he says, "I want my own doctor. . . . I'm interested in what's happening to me now, after these nodes." Ronald has had two episodes of lymphadenopathy (enlarged lymph nodes) of unknown etiology since 1977. Both of these episodes of enlarged nodes were accompanied by two additional symptoms: (1) a fatigue of dramatic proportions and (2) a tendency to bruise readily. The enlarged nodes were surgically removed after the first episode of lymphadenopathy, and Ronald remembers being told, simply enough, that he had "enlarged lymph nodes." At that time, his level of concern about his health was so minimal that he didn't even ask any further questions about his illness.

However, the second episode left Ronald somewhat more concerned about the state of his health. In the interim between the first and second episodes of lymphadenopathy, he had heard the newscaster Walter Cronkite announce the toll free number that the Department of Defense established for atomic veterans. He began to get a bit "leery" at that point, "but really hadn't thought about the fact that radiation can cause lymphoma and enlarged nodes until the second time around." At that point, he began to wonder if he had a radiogenic lymphoma. He went to a doctor, told him that he had been an atomic veteran, and generally expressed his concerns. His physician gave him antibiotics and the nodes returned to normal size within days. Ronald received tests for leukemia and Hodgkins Disease, and they turned out to be negative.

At the time of our interviews, Ronald had concluded that "I know that I am symptomatic. I know it's physical, but that I don't have cancer. It must be something else." He said that "probably every illness I get in the future will make me wonder." Then he corrected himself and said that "actually not every illness, only those illnesses I don't understand."

One further example of heightened concern about one's health in consequence of the belief that one's body has been damaged by an exposure to ionizing radiation comes from the work of Robert J. Lifton with the survivors of the bombing of Hiroshima. Lifton found both elements of the phenomenon that we have been discussing. He found survivors who believed that their bodies had been contaminated and damaged and he found this belief in association with patients' preoccupation with their health.

Among other similar cases, Lifton tells of a European priest who said that he had been exposed at Hiroshima to a dose of radiation large enough to have caused acute radiation sickness. At the time of Lifton's study (1962), this man complained of chronic exhaustion, dizziness, and a general inability to work. Even though he had been found by his physicians to have no demonstrable illness, this man told Lifton, "People [like us] become uneasy, because with no reason these things occur. Then three months after getting one thing, something of a new kind begins. Right now I am not normal. . . . You are always thinking: what is the next thing that will happen?"[8] Lifton found that the exposure to radiation often led survivors to believe that they had what he has called an "enduring taint; a taint of death which attaches itself not only to one's entire psychological organism, but through potential genetic defects to one's posterity as well."[9]

This sense of taint apparently gave rise in many of the *Hibakusha,* or atomic bomb survivors, to an intense preoccupation with their health. This preoccupation was of sufficient proportion among Hiroshima survivors to have been noticed and given a special diagnostic label by Hiroshima physicians. In Lifton's words: "Hiroshima doctors have another term, 'A-Bomb Neurosis,' which they apply to behavior that appears to be psychically caused, especially to those who become involved in a lifelong preoccupation with 'A-Bomb Disease—with blood counts and bodily complaints, particularly that of weakness—to the point of greatly restricting their lives or even becoming bedridden."[10]

The "A-Bomb Neurosis" is another example of a response to a radiation exposure in which there is an association between the belief that one's body has been damaged and a preoccupation with one's body and health. Several studies indicate that this type of association is not limited to radiation exposures.

Brodsky's work, for example, on the somatoform illnesses developed by workers occupationally exposed to toxic chemicals, is one of several studies that has demonstrated that this sense of damaged flesh accompanied by a heightened concern about the status of one's somatic health can also occur among people who have been exposed to toxic chemicals.[11] Brodsky describes the existence of two different groups of patients among his subjects, both of whom embarked upon illness careers subsequent to their occupational exposures to toxic chemicals. These patients were all involved, to Brodsky's eye, with illness careers in the sense that each of them had a prolonged history of vague and/or nonspecific somatic symptoms for which they had not been able to obtain medical diagnosis or treatment. Their lives became centered around the disabilities introduced into their existence by their symptoms and around obtaining diagnosis, treatment, and compensation for their illness. "Nearly half" of Brodsky's subjects were no longer working.

Their lives were characterized by the belief that they had been physically harmed by the chemicals to which they had been exposed. All seventy subjects "believed they had been injured by inhaling non-infectious, airborne substances in the workplace."[12] In turn, this belief led them to a pronounced concern with their health. Brodsky describes the several subgroups he found within his larger study group in the following ways:[13]

1. "They began to see themselves as fragile and weak."
2. "The event of toxic exposure, which all of them experienced, made them perceive themselves as damaged or impaired. Then they looked for physical and mental changes, and any perceived differences in hearing, vision, strength, stamina, memory or interests were attributed to exposure."
3. "The pre-morbid histories of this group showed recurring features: a long history of preoccupation and concern over personal health; recurring symptoms over many years; and multiple visits to physicians who find no objective basis for the subjective complaints."
4. "These subjects had a long history of concern and preoccupation with their bodies, a concern directed to risks in the external environment."

It seems safe to conclude that Brodsky has found among workers occupationally exposed to toxic chemicals the same conjunction that we have already seen in people who have been exposed to radiation: (1) a belief that their bodies have been contaminated and damaged by an invisible environmental contaminant and (2) a resultant preoccupation with and concern for their health. Reich[14] found much the same phenomena in all three of his case studies and both Levine[15] and Fowlkes and Miller[16] observed the same events in their studies of the Love Canal disaster.

The preoccupation with their health that develops in people who have been exposed to an invisible environmental contaminant is a form of hypervigilance. It is a form of hypervigilance in that it is a pattern of cognition and behavior, as defined by Janis, that is characterized by:[17]

1. An alertness to all signs of potential threat that results in a diffusion of attention
2. A strong motivation to engage in a thorough search and appraisal
3. Obsessional ideas about all the things that could go wrong
4. Indiscriminate attentiveness to all sorts of threats, both relevant and irrelevant.

As we determined earlier, hypervigilance can develop as a response to a threatening situation in which the threatened person realizes that the information needed to adapt successfully to the threat at hand will not be available. This is precisely the circumstance of the person who becomes ill after an exposure to an invisible contaminant. This is particularly true of the individual who has somatic symptoms that his or her physician cannot diagnose. For the person who believes that he or she has been or may have been injured by an invisible exposure, every new symptom or illness raises a plethora of new questions. For example:

1. The patient who has a cancer will want to know if it was caused by the invisible contaminant to which he or she was exposed.
2. The patient who has had a series of serious illnesses since an invisible exposure will want to know if the illnesses have been caused by that exposure.
3. The patient who has undiagnosed physical symptoms will want to know if those symptoms are the first as of yet unrecognizable signs of a serious illness caused by the contaminant to which he or she was exposed.
4. All of these patients will want to know if they will develop contaminant-caused illness in the future.
5. All of these patients will regard every new symptom with fear and suspicion, and they will want proof that these symptoms are not a manifestation of a contaminant-caused disease.

These questions are only the most salient and obvious of those that will arise. When it becomes evident to the exposed persons that these questions are unanswerable and that they are in a situation in which they can not be vigilant about the effects of a contamination on their health, hypervigilance will set in. As predicted by Janis's ambiguity hypothesis, these patients will intensify their search for the information they think they need to protect themselves. They will want this information in order to: (1) minimize the health effects of that previous exposure and (2) detect incipient contaminant-caused illness at the earliest possible juncture so as to insure the best possible medical outcome.

This hypervigilance is often misunderstood by physicians. They do not understand it as a hypertrophied and distorted version of a legitimate need to be vigilant about one's health. The tendency by physicians to diagnose patients who have been exposed to an invisible contaminant as being hypochondriacal has been documented in four populations that have been exposed to an invisible contaminant. They are as follows:

1. The Hiroshima survivors who were exposed to ionizing radiation[18]
2. Atomic veterans who were also exposed to ionizing radiation[19]
3. The residents of western Japan who were exposed to PCB present in their cooking oil[20]
4. Workers who have been occupationally exposed to a variety of toxic chemicals.[21]

Lifton reports that "studies have shown that Hibakusha are more generally prone to hypochondriasis than other people, especially those who experienced the symptoms of acute irradiation at the time of the bomb." He indicates that many survivors became preoccupied with their health and were regarded as being neurotic and hypochondriacal by Hiroshima physicians. Lifton was careful to note, however, that "as compared to usual hypochondriacal and phobic patterns encountered in psychiatric work, those in ['A-Bomb Neurosis'] are much more directly related to actual bodily assaults that can result from atomic bomb exposure."[22]

In my own work with atomic veterans, I have received an overwhelming number of reports from these men that their physicians almost invariably regarded them as hypochondriacs. The following dialogue exemplifies this aspect of the atomic veteran experience:

> —None of the doctors I've ever seen believed that any of my problems has been caused by radiation. But I'm going to prove it to them.
> —*How will that change things?*
> —Well, then they won't think I'm a hypochondriac, and they'll treat me with more respect. They'll start helping me more when I say I've got a radiation problem. They'll dig into it and find out what the problem is.[23]

Another veteran, who has seen by his own count twenty-three doctors in his search for diagnosis and treatment for his neuromuscular symptoms, had this to say about his relationship to physicians:

—The experience of being told that there is nothing wrong with me by a succession of twenty-three doctors has changed the way I talk to them.

—*How do you mean?*

—I used to go on at length and describe the history of my symptoms in detail. I thought that would help them make the diagnosis, but now I know what they're going to say, and I'm ashamed of being seen as a hypochondriac, so I say it all real quick and get it over with.

—*Why do you keep going back?*

—Because I know that this muscle weakness and pain is real; and that it has something to do with radiation; and that sooner or later, I'll find a doctor who will know what to do about it.[24]

A recurring theme among atomic veterans is that their physicians tell them that their problems are "all in your head." As one atomic veteran who gets his medical care from the Veterans Adminstration told me, "I think the Veterans Administration tags us atomic veterans as psychological problems. You have to be on the defense when you go to the Veterans Administration."

In the Japanese rice bran oil contamination, public health officials developed the perception that a number of people were overly and unnecessarily concerned about the personal effects of that PCB contamination. Officials thought that the contamination involved a large number of people because the contaminated cooking oil was a widely consumed product in western Japan. To determine how extensive the contamination was, the Ministry of Health and Welfare directed that all people with Yusho—the illness caused by the PCB contamination—register with public health centers. The number of people who registered reached 14,000. "Symptoms among these people ranged from severe to light. According to a ministry official, when doctors examined some registered cases of suspected poisoning in Fukuoka Prefecture, they found that 'unmistakable' Yusho patients represented only ten percent of the total. The majority, the official said, suffered from 'rice bran oil neurosis.'"[25]

A final example of a perceived hypochondriasis in those exposed to invisible contaminants is Brodsky's work on somatoform symptoms in workers occupationally exposed to toxic chemicals. Brodsky himself regards the somatic or physical complaints with which his seventy referred patients presented as being somatoform symptoms. That is, he regards them as "physical symptoms that suggest physical disorder (hence somatoform) but for which there are no demonstrable organic findings or known physiological mechanisms and for which there is positive evidence, or a strong presumption, that the symptoms are linked to psychological factors or conflicts. Unlike those in fictitious disorder or malingering, the symptoms in somatoform disorders are not under voluntary control, i.e., the individual does not experience the sense of controlling the symptoms."[26] In addition, Brodsky sees his subjects as exhibiting classical hypochondriacal behavior. To be more specific, he sees them as being entrenched in illness careers in which they are intensely preoccupied with their health.

Thus in his study Brodsky is not reporting on a situation in which physicians have implicitly or explicitly diagnosed individuals exposed to an invisible environmental contaminant as being hypochondriacs. He has actually taken that position himself. He presents us with seventy exposed patients whom he regards as having somatoform and hypochondriacal symptoms. Although the perspective is somewhat different, the import of Brodsky's work is that it provides further documentation of the fact that people exposed to the invisible contaminants are often regarded as hypochondriacs by the physicians that they see.

I would like to quickly state that I will be taking issue at a later point in this chapter with both the theoretical and clinical positions that Dr. Brodsky's approach represents. In particular, I will take issue with Dr. Brodsky's assertion that the illness careers that his subjects brought to his office are primarily a manifestation of preexisting psychological conflicts that they had brought with them into the toxic workplace. Preexisting conflicts may well have played some role in the genesis of the illness careers that Dr. Brodsky described, but the weight of the evidence considered in this book suggests that the hypervigilant response to an invisible exposure, of which the illness career is an example, must be regarded as a recurring psychological consequence of the exposure to an invisible contaminant. Dr. Brodsky does not seem to have considered this hypothesis, and the resulting difference in perspective is of considerable theoretical and clinical import.

Before looking at the full spectrum of issues raised by this diagnosis in an invisible exposure, I would like to first summarize the sequence of events described in this chapter. These events can be schematically represented as shown in figure 16–1.

The figure expresses the following dynamic: some of the people who are exposed to an invisible environmental contaminant will either become concerned about whether that exposure has biologically harmed them, or they will actually become convinced that it has harmed them. Either circumstance will lead a person to want to become vigilant about the health effects of that exposure. In the process of going to their physicians with their concerns, the exposed people learn that neither they nor their physicians will be able to generate the information that will be needed to maintain that vigilance successfully. Hypervigilance about their health is the result, as predicted by the ambiguity hypothesis. In turn, this hypervigilance is perceived and diagnosed as hypochondriasis by their physicians. Finally, the diagram raises the question of whether the hypervigilance process itself might generate somatoform symptoms. Unfortunately there are not sufficient data with which to answer this question at this time.

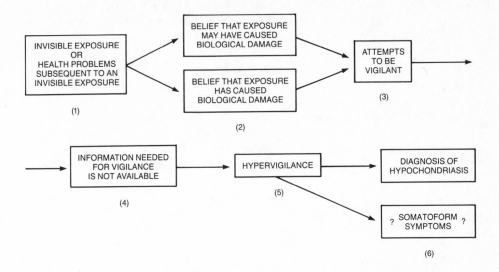

Figure 16–1. Medical Dysfunction

As indicated in the diagram, the hypervigilant response to an invisible exposure is a consequence of believing that one has been or may have been injured by that exposure. These beliefs are usually precipitated by some kind of evidence that suggests to the exposee that a contaminant-caused injury has occurred. In most cases, this evidence takes the form of medical problems subsequent to an invisible exposure. The priest who survived the bombing of Hiroshima had acute radiation sickness immediately after the blast.[27] The Love Canal families who believed that the canal posed a serious threat to their health were the families whose members had suffered from recurrent and chronic somatic symptoms that their physicians were unable to diagnose.[28] The atomic veterans who were preoccupied with their health and who believed that they had been injured by radiation were characteristically men who had one of three types of postexposure medical histories: (1) cancer, (2) a sequence of several major medical problems, or (3) undiagnosable somatic symptoms.[29]

Despite the varied nature of the medical problems that can generate a vigilant and eventually hypervigilant patient, it seems that the undiagnosable somatic symptoms cause the most concern for a person who has been exposed to an invisible contaminant. Somatic symptoms for which a diagnosis cannot be obtained create a lack of closure that can be virtually unbearable for the exposed person. Undiagnosable symptoms forcefully raise the possibility in the exposed person's mind that his or her symptoms are the first sign of a contaminant-caused disease that physicians have not yet recognized.

Until diagnosed, these symptoms become a constant reminder that some kind of terrible contaminant-caused illness may well be gestating in the exposed person's body.

This notion is particularly difficult to dismiss when the undiagnosed symptom or symptoms persist. Their persistence amplifies their threatening quality and reinforces the notion that they are in fact the manifestation of an as-yet-undetected contaminant-caused illness. Not even the considered opinion of a doctor that the symptom is "all in your head" will persuade the exposed person to relinquish his or her concerns. In fact, the diagnosis of hypochondriasis has a curious paradoxical effect upon the exposed person with undiagnosed symptoms: it strengthens his or her conviction that the symptoms are an expression of a contaminant-caused disease, and at the same time it makes the person wonder if maybe he or she is somehow imagining the whole thing. John, the atomic veteran who saw eleven doctors before receiving a diagnosis of dermatomyositis for his neuromuscular symptoms, said, "I was beginning to wonder if I was crazy "

This convergence of invisible exposures and hypervigilance in patients who have undiagnosed somatic symptoms has been noted over and over again. Lifton has described the preoccupations and undiagnosable symptoms of the Hiroshima survivors.[30] Brodsky has written about the illness careers and somatoform symptoms of workers occupationally exposed to toxic chemicals.[31] Fowlkes and Miller have been extremely interested in the incentive qualities of the undiagnosable symptoms found among residents of the Love Canal neighborhood. They also took note of the difficulties such people had in obtaining medical care for those symptoms.[32] Reich described, in careful depth, the dysfunctional psychological impacts of undiagnosed contaminant-caused symptoms in all three of his case studies. He found hypervigilance, preoccupation, and distress in consequence of a PBB contamination in Michigan, PCB contamination in Japan, and a dioxin contamination in Italy.[33] Finally, I have reported on the appearance of undiagnosable symptoms and health preoccupations among the atomic veterans.[34]

Given the constant and recurring appearance of undiagnosable symptoms among individuals exposed to the invisible contaminants and, given the importance that these symptoms come to have in their lives, it becomes essential to ask the following questions: Why do these undiagnosable symptoms characteristically develop among individuals who have been exposed to the invisible contaminants? What are the causes of these symptoms? Are they somatoform symptoms? Or are they somatic symptoms caused by the invisible exposure in question?

First, let us note that there is a definite association between invisible exposures and hypervigilant behavior and undiagnosed symptoms in exposed people. This suggests that there may be a causal relationship between invisible exposures and the latter two phenomena, and that any hypothesis regarding the causation of the undiagnosable symptoms would have to take these facts into account. It also suggests that there may be some relationship between the hypervigilant behavior and the appearance of undiagnosable symptoms in exposed individuals. However, before considering this possibility, I would like to consider two questions: (1) What is the relationship between invisible exposures and subsequent exposee preoccupations with the health effects of that exposure? (2) What is the nature of the relationship between invisible exposures and the undiagnosable symptoms with which exposed individuals present to their physicians?

The first question is relatively easy to answer. The medical preoccupations of the person who has been exposed to an invisible contaminant are a form of hypervigilance. They are the end product of a frustrated and distorted attempt to maintain vigilance over the possible health effects of an invisible exposure. They are the result of attempts to adapt to the threats posed by an invisible contamination; attempts that failed because the information needed to adapt to those threats was not available. As such, these preoccupations are clearly a psychological response to an invisible exposure.

The second question is much more difficult. It is complicated by the mind–body problem and the uncertain nature of the symptoms themselves. Basically, there are two possible theoretical explanations for the origins of these undiagnosable symptoms:

1. They are somatic symptoms that are an expression of an as-yet-unrecognized somatic illness caused by the contaminant in question, or

2. They are somatoform symptoms that appear to be of a physical nature to both patient and physican but that have no organic component at all.

The somatoform hypothesis itself can take three forms:

1. The somatoform symptoms are caused solely by psychological conflicts that the exposed person had before exposure to the invisible contaminant in question,

2. The somatoform symptoms are caused solely by psychological conflicts that result from the invisible exposure that the patient has experienced, or

3. The somatoform symptoms are caused by an interaction between a person's preexisting conflicts and the psychological stresses generated by an invisible exposure. More specifically, the dilemmas generated by an invisible exposure make manifest preexisting conflicts that are already present in the exposed individual.

Of these three somatoform hypotheses, it is a simple task to eliminate the first one. The data at which we have been looking clearly indicate that there is an association between invisible exposures and somatic/somatoform symptoms, and that the invisible exposures themselves somehow play a role in causing these symptoms. To hold to the somatoform hypothesis is to ignore the strength of the findings on this association.

In addition, as both Brodsky and I have observed, the somatic/somatoform symptoms are part of the same fabric in which the health preoccupations are woven. The observed preoccupations concern the undiagnosable symptoms. The illness careers of Dr. Brodsky's patients were centered around the somatoform symptoms present in those patients. These symptoms appear, in fact, to somehow be a part of the hypervigilance that appears in response to an invisible exposure. One additional piece of evidence suggests that the symptoms are related to the invisible exposures: the finding that the prevalence of hypochondriasis was elevated among survivors of the bombing of Hiroshima. Thus it seems entirely appropriate to eliminate the first somatoform hypothesis.

On the other hand, despite the strong observed association between invisible exposures and the appearance of undiagnosable symptoms, it is not possible to eliminate the third, or interaction, hypothesis. After all, not everyone who is exposed to an invisible contaminant goes on to develop this type of symptomatology. Something else must be at work. In addition, Dr. Brodsky's study seems to indicate that preexisting material can be found in patients who have developed somatoform symptoms. Nonetheless, data that would permit us to eliminate either the second or third somatoform hypotheses do not exist. Longitudinal studies of exposed cohorts, starting from the time of exposure, and additional studies of the prevalence of undiagnosable/somatoform symptoms in exposed populations would be of help here.

Regardless of which of the remaining somatoform hypotheses is correct, it can be seen that both the undiagnosable symptoms and the hypervigilant process are a response to the occurrence of an invisible exposure. This means that we are basically left with two hypotheses about the etiology of the somatic/somatoform symptoms seen in the wake of an invisible exposure:

1. They are undiagnosable somatic symptoms that are the expression of an as-yet-unrecognized somatic illness caused by the contaminant in question, or

2. They are somatoform symptoms that have developed as a psychological response to the dilemmas posed by an invisible exposure. (It remains an open question as to what role preexisting conflicts play in the development of these symptoms.)

I would like to consider, at this point, the clinical implications of both of these hypotheses. Suppose for a moment that you are a physician seeing a patient who has been exposed to an invisible contaminant, and that the patient has presented to you with both undiagnosable symptoms and with evident concerns about the health effects of that exposure. The patient was exposed to radiation twelve years ago and is now complaining of weakness and muscle pain in both legs. In addition, the patient had a skin cancer removed from his face two years ago.

You cannot decide for certain whether the symptoms with which he is now presenting are of a somatic or somatoform nature. On the one hand, you have found some minor abnormalities on physical examination. The deep tendon reflexes in the right leg seem to be a bit sluggish, and a nerve conduction study of the same leg shows that his conduction rates are at the bottom end of the normal range. However, you cannot make a diagnosis, or even determine for certain whether the patient's symptoms are a consequence of a somatic process. Nonetheless, you cannot dismiss the possibility.

Your situation is complicated by the fact that you have worked with a number of patients who have been exposed to radiation. You have become aware that medical knowledge about the health effects of radiation has been in constant flux and evolution since the discovery of ionizing radiation in 1896. It took forty years for science to recognize that exposure to radiation could cause cancers and birth defects at doses that did not cause the acute and observable health effects of radiation exposure. It took another fifteen years to discover that radiation could cause cataracts. In addition, animal studies have demonstrated that radiation can cause a full range of nontumorous diseases that have yet to be found among human beings. It seems entirely possible to you that radiation may cause other illnesses that have not yet been recognized by medical research.

Now suppose that you decide that your patient's symptoms are somatic symptoms of an illness that is not yet sufficiently manifest or understood to make diagnosis of these symptoms possible. Given that you are uncertain about the diagnosis, how can you best pursue the evaluation of those symptoms and, at the same time, minimize the possibility that your patient will develop adverse psychological effects of exposure to an invisible contaminant? The question, in terms of the stress and coping model, is this: Given that neither you nor your patient has sufficient information with which to make the usual medical adaptations of diagnosis and treatment to your patient's symptoms, how can you relate to this patient and his illness so as to reduce to an absolute minimum the amount of adaptational failure that he will experience in trying to adapt to the health effects of an invisible exposure? As we have already seen, it is these failures, for the most part attributable to the medical invisibility of a contaminant, that generate the adverse psychological effects of that exposure.

For the patients who want to maintain careful vigilance over the health effects of an invisible exposure, the primary source of avoidable adaptational failure is the discovery that their physicians are not as concerned as they are with maintaining vigilance over the effects of that exposure. If their physicians are not as concerned as they are, then patients cannot mount the level of vigilance that they would like to maintain. For patients to maintain vigilance, they must depend on the knowledge and capacities of their physicians. In other words, they can't do it alone; they need their physicians' assistance in this task.

The greatest concern and fear for patients in this position is that their physicians, in finding no visible evidence of contaminant-caused illness, might reach any of the following categorical conclusions: (1) no contaminant-caused disease is present, (2) no contaminant-caused disease will appear in the future, and (3) it is not necessary to maintain persistent vigilance over the potential health effects of a past invisible exposure. Patients become either implicitly or explicitly aware of medical invisibility, and consequently they become aware of the possibility that their physicians might prematurely dismiss their concerns because there is no manifest evidence of contaminant-caused disease.

This, then, is the central problem and source of adaptational failure for a patient who has been exposed to an invisible contaminant. The most important and reassuring thing for exposed and vigilant patients is to be able to believe that their physicians are (1) genuinely concerned about the health effects of the contaminant to which they were exposed and (2) both understanding and respectful of the patients' needs to maintain careful vigilance over the potential health effects of that exposure. If patients are unable to find such physicians, their fears and concerns about their health will be amplified, and they will feel ashamed of and diminished in their concerns about their health.

The cardinal rule, then, for physicians seeing patients who have a history of invisible exposure, is to recognize that many of them will have a somewhat hypertrophied need to monitor the health effects of that exposure. It is important for physicians to communicate that they understand their patients' vigilance needs. Tell your patient that you are aware of the medical invisibility of the contaminant to which he or she has been exposed, and of the difficulties that this invisibility imposes on the process of diagnosing and treating the illnesses caused by the contaminant. Let the patient know that you will not be misled by the invisibility of the contaminant, and that you will not assume, because you have yet to find evidence of illness or contamination, that the contaminant *has* or *has not* affected the patient's health. Let the patient know that you will continue to monitor his or her health carefully.

In addition, it will be helpful to take the time to involve such patients in your own thinking about their health. This approach will enhance patients' feeling that they are successfully monitoring their health. Be impeccably honest. Tell patients what you do know and what you do not know about the health effects of the contamination that they have endured. Admit when you are uncertain about something, perhaps the diagnosis of a particular symptom, and explain why you are uncertain. Be careful, in your own mind, that the statements you make to exposed patients about their health are based on observation and not on speculation or assumption.

An important consequence of taking this approach is that it encourages exposed patients to remain open-minded about the potential health effects of a previous invisible exposure. This is one of the most important things that physicians can do to *prevent* the development of preoccupation and trauma in their exposed patients. If an exposed patient is not convinced that he or she will be the subject of concerned medical vigilance that takes into account the medical invisibility of a contaminant, there is a good chance that the patient will mount his or her own vigilance campaign and decide, in support of that campaign, that something is definitely or probably wrong with his or her health. From this decision or belief proceeds the hypervigilance, preoccupation, and psychological trauma of an invisible exposure. Thus one of the important goals of medical care for exposed patients is to encourage them to remain open-minded about the health effects of an exposure until the accumulated evidence indicates what belief is appropriate.

Perhaps the single most efficient method that physicians have for convincing their exposed patients that they do not share their concerns about an invisible exposure is to tell those patients that they are hypochondriacs; that their needs for vigilance are overwrought, and that their symptoms are "all in your head." Such an approach not only places patients in a quandary as to how they can best monitor their health, it also leaves them feeling ashamed of their concerns and, if their symptoms persist, doubting their own sanity.

So what, then, does one do, as a physician, when confronted with an exposed patient whose undiagnosable symptoms are somatoform symptoms? What does one do when it becomes evident that a patient's symptoms have a psychogenic origin that is somehow related to his or her exposure to an invisible environmental contaminant? How can one respond to such patients in such a way as to minimize the likelihood that they will develop the adverse psychological effects of exposure?

The basic answer would seem to be one of taking the same approach that one would take with the exposed patient whose undiagnosable symptoms are somatic. The reason for taking this approach is as follows: Both patients are facing the same adaptational dilemmas. Both patients are concerned with monitoring the health effects of an invisible exposure. Both are confronted with the problem of coping with threats to their health in the absence of the kind of information that their physicians need to adapt successfully to those threats.

The difference between the two patients, if our clinical judgments about the nature of their symptoms has been correct, lies in the etiology of their undiagnosable symptoms. One patient's symptoms have a somatic origin, and the second patient's symptoms are probably a manifestation of the traumatic psychological consequences of his or her exposure to an invisible contaminant. One must still say "probably," because at this point it is only a hypothesis that the somatoform symptoms are a psychological consequence of an exposure to an invisible contaminant. It is true that the occurrence of hypochondriasis is a constant finding in the wake of an invisible exposure, but the mechanism by which such symptoms are produced is not known.

Both patients are faced with the adaptational dilemmas posed by an invisible exposure, and it seems possible that the patient with somatoform symptoms has developed those symptoms as a part of his or her psychological response to the exposure. The task of the physician seeing this second type of patient is to help that patient adapt to the exposure and gain a sense of control and vigilance over the potential health effects of that exposure.

In summary, then, the clinical approach to a patient who has been exposed to an invisible contaminant must be tempered with a knowledge of the traumatic psychological effects of those contaminants. The medical care given to the exposed patient should have, among its goals, the prevention and/or treatment of the potential or actual psychological traumata of an invisible exposure. The basic approach to the exposed patient with or without somatoform symptoms is to create a situation in which that patient will not feel the need to become hypervigilant about the previous exposure. The basic means by which this goal is accomplished is by recognizing and addressing the vigilance needs of the exposed patient.

Unfortunately, most exposed patients are seen by physicians who are not familiar with the psychology of the invisible contaminants. This is understandable; research into the psychological effects of the invisible environmental contaminants is still in a nascent stage. As a result, it often seems to be the case that patients who have been exposed to an invisible contaminant do not receive medical care that addresses their psychological dilemmas and needs. One indication of this is the frequency with which such patients are told that they are hypochondriacs. The patient whose hypervigilance is diagnosed and treated as hypochondriasis is probably not receiving help with the tasks of vigilance.

Another effect, as we have already seen, of telling a patient that he or she is a hypochondriac is that it spurs the patient on to even greater heights of hypervigilance. The diagnosis of hypochondriasis tells the patient that the physician will not take seriously patient concerns about the health effects of a previous contamination. This increases the patient's drive to fend for himself or herself and/or find other more helpful physicians. The diagnosis of hypochondriasis becomes part of a positive feedback cycle in which the exposed patient becomes increasingly vigilant and afraid for his or her health. One has to see such patients to comprehend the fevered pitch into which they can be thrown.

Ultimately, the exposed patients who are seen by physicians that do not understand the psychology of the invisible contaminants will grow increasingly discontent. They will conclude that those physicians don't comprehend anything about the somatic effects of the involved contaminant. They will conclude that they have contaminant-caused illnesses that their physicians cannot diagnose. They will also become ashamed of being seen as hypochondriacs. After seeing ten or twenty doctors who can't seem to help them with their problems, they will begin to wonder if maybe they are crazy. All of this is unnecessary and avoidable.

The ground of the dysfunctional dynamic that develops between doctors and exposed patients is the result of a difference in conception between doctor and patient of the doctor's role in treating such a contamination. Most physicians take the medical role that they have been trained to take. They detect, diagnose, and treat illnesses that have already become clinically apparent. This can be called the treatment approach to medicine, and in many clinical situations it is an adequate and good approach to take.

However, in many instances, including clinical situations that involve exposed patients who are concerned about the health effects of a previous contamination, the treatment approach is not enough. In the case of the contaminated patient, this is not an appropriate approach because the patient has legitimate needs for his physician to take what can be called a preventive vigilance approach.

As we have already seen, the exposed patients who are concerned about their health want to be vigilant about the potential health effects of that exposure. They believe that contaminant-caused illness may be gestating within their bodies, and that the proper medical approach to their health is to keep eyes constantly peeled for the first signs of this illness. Their belief is that early detection is their best hope for preventing the full development of the contaminant-caused illnesses. This is why they want their physicians to take a preventive vigilance approach to their medical care, and it is exactly this approach that many exposed patients feel they are not receiving from their physicians.

It is this difference in conception of physicians' roles that leads to the development of dysfunctional relationships. Physicians take a treatment approach, and patients want their physicians to take a preventive vigilance approach. The resultant discrepancy in expectations often leaves the exposed patients feeling bitterly discontent with their medical care.

A definition, then, of a dysfunctional medical relationship (DMR) is as follows: A DMR is a relationship between a physician and a patient exposed to an invisible environmental contaminant in which: (1) the patient feels that many of his or her important medical needs are not being addressed and (2) the physician's approach to the patient is exacerbating the adverse psychological effects of the invisible contaminants. The cause of this dysfunction is a difference in conception between doctor and patient as to what the doctor's proper functions should be in relating to a patient who has been exposed to an invisible contaminant. As we shall be seeing in the next chapter, DMRs can take more than one form.

death that occurred in 1953 and (b) an increased rate of childhood leukemia in the downwind areas of Utah.[2]

3. At Love Canal, a still-unresolved dispute arose as to whether the chemicals released from the canal were causing illness among residents of the area.[3]

4. In Michigan, a still-unresolved conflict arose as to whether the PBB contamination of livestock feed resulted in (a) livestock illness and (b) human illness.[4]

5. In the Japanese PCB contamination of rice bran cooking oil, the controversy as to whether that contamination caused human illness has never been resolved.[5]

6. The use of the herbicide Agent Orange in Vietnam by the U.S. military forces raised the as-yet-unresolved question of whether that herbicide caused cancers and birth defects in the Vietnamese and U.S. military populations.[6]

7. The atmospheric testing of nuclear weapons has raised unresolved questions of whether military participants in these tests, the atomic veterans, have developed a large spectrum of illnesses as a result of their exposure to radiation.[7]

8. The Bhopal accident in India has spawned a vast array of controversies about the health effects of the accident. These unresolved controversies include the issues of what chemicals were actually released from the plant, whether those chemicals have caused chronic illness in the Bhopal area, and what methods of treatment should be used to treat the resulting illnesses.[8]

9. Finally, the ongoing occupational exposure of workers to invisible contaminants constantly raises the question of whether their illnesses have been caused by those exposures.[9]

This list indicates that not only are conflicts about the health effects of an invisible exposure a frequent component of such exposures, but that it is most often the case that such conflicts are never resolved.

These conflicts are usually initiated when an exposed individual or group of individuals claims that they have become ill as a result of the exposure. Conflicts can also begin with exposee requests for termination or alteration of the contamination-producing technologies with which they live or work. In making these claims, exposed people are usually seeking either: (1) medical care for their illnesses, (2) measures that will arrest all further exposure to a contaminant (for example, government purchase of housing at Love Canal), or (3) financial compensation for the unwanted changes brought into their lives by the exposure in question.

17
Blaming the Victim Twice

I f the primary currency of an invisible exposure is uncertainty, the seco
ary currency is blame. The question invariably arises in the wake
significant exposure as to whether that particular exposure has cau
the illnesses that subsequently develop in the exposed population. The in
tutions responsible for the contamination tend to claim that the cont
ination has not caused subsequent illness. On the other hand, many of
exposed people who become ill will contend that the contamination in qu
tion has caused their illness. The situation is complicated by the fact that
medical invisibility of the involved contaminants—particularly their etiol
ical invisibility—makes it almost impossible to resolve the question of cau
tion in an empirical manner.

The result is often a protracted conflict about the causes of the illness
question. The resulting dialogue takes on, most often, a political as oppo
to a scientific character. It is part of the nature of these dialogues that
participating parties trade accusations of responsibility and blame betwe
themselves. This chapter looks at the manner in which this dialogue abo
responsibility and blame affects the perception of the psychological effects
exposures to these invisible environmental contaminants.

Conflicts about the health effects of specific exposures to the invisib
contaminants have become part of the landscape in the second half of t
twentieth century. Just to remind ourselves of the central place that these co
flicts hold in our lives, I would like to list some of the better known occasio
on which these conflicts have arisen:

1. In consequence of the Three Mile Island accident, arguments ha
   already arisen as to whether the radiation released by that accident h
   caused (a) an increased incidence of livestock illness and (b) an increase
   incidence of neonatal hypothyroidism and infant death in human beings

2. In consequence of the atmospheric testing of nuclear weapons at th
   Nevada Test Site, conflicts have arisen as to whether the radiatio
   released by those tests has caused (a) the excessive amount of livestoc

In each of the contaminations listed above, the involved institutions have in general contended that the illnesses in question were not caused by the associated contamination. The Atomic Energy Commission took the adamant position that the Utah livestock deaths had not been caused by radiation.[10] The Nuclear Regulatory Commission held, years later, that the livestock illness at Three Mile Island had not been caused by the accident there. The Pennsylvania Department of Health claimed that there was no increase in neonatal hypothyroidism or infant deaths after Three Mile Island. The Department of Defense has claimed that Agent Orange does not cause cancers and birth defects.[11] The Veterans Administration holds that the vast majority of the atomic veterans do not have radiogenic illness. Of the more than atomic veterans who have applied for service-related benefits, only fourteen have been judged by the Veterans Administration to be eligible for such benefits.[12] Farm Bureau Services claimed that Michigan dairy herd illness was unrelated to PBB contamination of their feed.[13]

One of the several approaches that the contaminating institutions have taken in contesting claims of contaminant-caused illness is to blame the exposed persons for the illnesses that they or their livestock have developed. This tactic seems to be part of the climate of blame and counterblame that grows up around the occurrence of an invisible exposure. For example, as related in chapter 6, Rick Halbert was told several times that his dairy herd's illness was probably due to some sort of error on his part.

Other farmers whose cattle were contaminated with PBBs were also blamed for livestock illness. They were blamed both before and after it became evident that an invisible exposure had occurred. In the first instance, farmers were blamed for the livestock illness by employees of the feed company. In the second instance, the farmers were blamed by "bureaucrats" working for state agencies.[14]

Blaming the victim has also occurred in situations involving an association between human illness and an invisible contamination. Most typically, blaming the victim develops as a response to a patient's hypervigilance and/or undiagnosable symptoms. In both cases, the attribution of blame takes the form of an implicit or explicit diagnosis of hypochondriasis. Once again, the blame occurs both before and after it becomes known that an invisible contamination has taken place.

In the case of the Kamino family, who live on the western Japanese island of Kyushu, the blame for their illness was subtle, and it developed in response to their undiagnosable symptoms. Unknown to them, or anyone else, the family was consuming rice bran cooking oil that was contaminated with PCB. In March 1968 family members became symptomatic as a result of the contamination. Their symptoms were most often nonspecific and vague, and included: loss of appetite, fatigue, excessive perspiration, swollen eyelids and extremities, headaches, weight loss, glue-like ocular secretions, loss of visual acuity at distances greater than five meters, and the eruption of acne-like boils over their entire bodies.

When the symptoms first appeared, the Kamino family attempted to treat them on their own. To no avail, they applied both Western medications and Chinese herbs. They then began to seek help from physicians. This, too, was not of any help. "Kamino sensed that if the doctors could not name the disease, then the patient must somehow be at fault."[15]

Fowlkes and Miller, in their study of Love Canal families, found the repeated and more explicit occurrence of blaming the victim. Again, the process of assigning blame to the victim developed in response to the appearance of undiagnosable symptoms:

> Overwhelmingly . . . persons who shared the belief that chemical migration was widespread also reported a constellation of health problems for which traditional medicine frequently has neither name nor specifically effective control or treatment over time. . . . Such residents received little support for their claims from either their own medical practitioners or from [public] health professionals charged with assessing the health effects of the leachate. Recall that all of the "believer" families recounted impressively similar [medical] histories with medical practitioners who were unable to locate [their] presenting symptoms [as] identifiable disease entities. Instead, their ailments were redefined as psychiatric or emotional in origin with the effect of "blaming the victim" for the sources as well as the manifestations of their problems. Many other residents reported these kinds of experiences with their doctors.[16]

In analogy to the Michigan contamination, the Love Canal residents were blamed for their symptoms by private physicians as well as by public health physicians working for the state Department of Health.

The atomic veterans have also been blamed for their medical problems by being diagnosed as hypochondriacs.[17] In their case, this assignation of blame developed as a response to both (1) their hypervigilant concerns about the effects of radiation on their health and (2) their undiagnosable symptoms. They received this response from their private physicians and especially from the staff physicians at the Veterans Administration hospitals, where atomic veterans who voiced their concern about radiation were often referred for psychiatric evaluation and treatment.

The following dialogue comes from an interview with an atomic veteran who died of leukemia and who had, prior to his diagnosis, recurrent difficulty in getting the Veterans Administration to regard his health problems as being of a somatic nature:

> —The one thing I'm really scared of is VA hospitals and doctors.
> —*Why?*

—They're controlled by the government, and the government is trying to suppress atomic survivors. The last time I was there one of the staff told me that he knew all about us atomic veterans. He said, "Oh, you're one of those guys. It's all in your head."[18]

The constant experience of atomic veterans has been one of discontent with the Veterans Administration. Such veterans feel that the Veterans Administration does not give them adequate medical care and compensation because the administration is constrained by government policy regarding the health effects of radiation. One atomic veteran, discussing the Veterans Administration's response to his attempts to prove that his medical problems were caused by radiation, said: "I have the feeling that the VA doctors are sympathetic, but that the administration won't allow them to speak their mind. The result is that the doctors are generally noncommittal. This is the feeling that most vets have. The doctors won't commit themselves, for example, to saying that my cataracts were caused by radiation. It would have eased my anxiety a lot to find out that the radiation caused my cataracts."[19]

The conflict that arises between atomic veterans and the Veterans Administration seems to be another example of the dialogue about responsibility and blame that inevitably occurs in the wake of an invisible exposure. These conflicts arise because much is at stake. For the institutions that are responsible for an exposure, great sums of money, their ability to continue their business and policies, and often their continued existence are at stake. For the exposed individual, health, the quality of life, and financial standing lie in the balance.

It is within the confines of this conflicted arena that the traumatic psychological effects of the invisible environmental contaminants make their vexed appearance. The conflicted situations that develop in consequence of an invisible exposure become one of the principal contexts within which these psychological traumas take on meaning. It seems true, but unfortunate, that this political dialogue ends up shaping the perceptions that the various parties to the conflict have of those psychological traumas.

Experience has shown that when evidence of the psychological effects of an invisible exposure is thrown into the midst of a dialogue about responsibility and blame, two things happen:

1. The institutions and individuals who have taken the position that the contamination in question is not the cause of the associated illness tend to point to the psychological problems caused by an exposure as evidence that the disputed somatic problems are all products of the exposed person's imagination. That is, they see such traumas as proof that the somatic illness in question has an emotional cause and is not physically related to the disputed contamination. Thus, the occurrence of the

trauma becomes yet another occasion on which the exposees are blamed for their illnesses.

2. As a result, the exposed individuals often come to be suspicious of any mention of the psychological trauma associated with an invisible exposure. They regard such discussion as an attempt to discredit their claims that their illnesses are organic diseases caused by the contaminant to which they have been exposed.

Herein lies the second layer of blame. The mental state of the individuals exposed to an invisible environmental contaminant becomes just another item in the political debate about the health effects of that exposure.

When one adds to this conflict dynamic the fact that our culture teaches a person to regard psychological problems and pathology as being his or her own fault, it becomes all too easy for exposees to become ashamed of their contaminant-caused psychological problems. Under these circumstances, their concerns about their health and their undiagnosable symptoms become, for them, a sign of weakness and an indication that their somatic problems are really unrelated to the contaminant to which they have been exposed.

In other words, the combined circumstances of contamination and culture work together to encourage the exposed person to (1) deny the psychological effects of an exposure and (2) be ashamed of those effects whenever they become evident. Neither of these developments is healthy or desirable. As we have already noted, the shame becomes an additional problem for the exposed person, and the denial prevents that person from taking on the necessary task of coming to terms with the problems.

It is important to state clearly that the mental states of people exposed to an invisible environmental contaminant should not be regarded as so many pawns in the political disputes that arise concerning the health effects of an exposure. Such a view is not empirically correct, and it damages the exposed individuals.

An implied empirical hypothesis is contained in the political positions taken in regard to the psychological effects of an invisible exposure. The hypothesis is this: the presence in an exposed individual of any of the adverse psychological effects of an invisible exposure indicates that the exposed person's somatic problems have a psychogenic origin. This hypothesis is incorrect. Studies have shown that people suffering from the psychological traumata of an invisible exposure fall into two categories. Some of them have genuine somatic illness that may well have been caused by a prior contamination,[20] while some of them appear to have somatoform symptoms that bear no physical relationship to the exposure in question.[21]

Thus it is accurate to say that sometimes the presence of psychological trauma indicates that a person's somatic complaints have a psychogenic origin and that sometimes they do not. Categorical statements to the contrary are simply incorrect. Furthermore, if exposed people are actually experiencing the psychological trauma of an invisible exposure, telling them that they are hypochondriacs will only make matters worse for them. The appropriate approach would be, once again, to address their needs for vigilance about the health effects of the invisible contaminant to which they have been exposed.

To blame exposed people for the psychological trauma that they have incurred in consequence of an invisible exposure only encourages them to deny and be ashamed of that trauma. Statements that blame exposees for their somatic illnesses are sometimes best understood as politically motivated statements occurring in the midst of a political dialogue about responsibility. When this occurs, they are probably an attempt by the person or institution making the statement to claim that they themselves are not responsible for the illness and/or trauma in question.

It would seem best, as a matter of clarity and accuracy, for the parties participating in an exposure conflict to remember that attempts to blame the victim are most often empirically incorrect. They are usually made in circumstances of empirical uncertainty and they are made as an attempt to preemptively divest one's self or institution of blame and/or responsibility for the health effects of an exposure. It goes without saying that this approach is not the best one for developing ethical resolutions to the difficult empirical questions that arise regarding responsibility for the illnesses and psychological trauma that develop subsequent to an invisible exposure.

18
The Institutional Denial of Invisible Threat

I n an article entitled "Hazard Visibility and Occupational Health Problem Solving: The Case of the Uranium Industry," Jessica Pearson presents a case study of institutional responses to the health threats posed by an invisible environmental contaminant.[1] In Pearson's words, her study "traces the history of government regulatory agency and industry response to the hazard of excessive mine radiation and the uranium industry in Colorado some thirty years ago." She is particularly interested in how the visibility or invisibility of a health hazard affects the institutional response to that hazard.

There was no uranium mining industry in the United States until the 1940s. The industry was actually created by the Atomic Energy Commission for the purpose of providing a domestic source of uranium for the production of nuclear weapons. Prior to the existence of the American industry, uranium mines had long been in operation in regions of what is today Czechoslovakia and East Germany. For centuries, it had been well known that miners working in these European uranium mines were particularly prone to die of a disease known as *Bergsucht*. By the late nineteenth century this disease had been identified as lung cancer. By 1933 lung cancer had been recognized as an occupational disease of miners.[2] Subsequent studies demonstrated that these radiogenic lung cancers were of two primary cell types: (1) oat cell carcinoma and (2) epidermoid carcinoma. We now know that these cancers are caused by the inhalation of a radioactive gas known as radon, which is released in large quantities by the process of mining for uranium.

Pearson tells us that "a number of studies of European uranium miners, during the late 1920s and early 1930s, were published in American journals; this research strongly suggested that radiation in mines was harmful to workers. American health officials were aware of the findings when the Atomic Energy Commission first declared its intention to stimulate a domestic uranium potential in 1947."[3] A remedy for the problem of radiation in mines had already been devised: a relatively simple and inexpensive method of removing radioactive air from uranium mines was developed in Czechoslovakia in the early 1950s. Machines were used to remove contaminated air from the mines and to replace it with fresh air.

Nonetheless, neither the Colorado mining industry nor the federal government took serious or systematic steps to prevent the development of radiogenic lung cancers in American miners until twenty years after the appearance of the American industry. In 1967, then Secretary of Labor Willard Wirtz invoked an existing piece of legislation (the Walsh Healy Contracts Act) to compel the enforcement of a uniform radiation standard in American uranium mines.

This sequence of events led Pearson to the following analysis and question:

> Today historians widely acknowledge that Wirtz's controversial action was a critical factor in the reduction of radiation in mines. This action, however, came a full twenty years after the Atomic Energy Commission had first sampled mines in an industry which it had created and found them at exposure levels comparable to those of the ill-fated mines of central Europe. The action came almost eighteen years after the first recorded discussions among officials in government agencies of possible radiation hazards in uranium mines. Moreover, nationwide control lagged seven years behind statistical documentation by the Public Health Service that uranium miners suffered elevated mortality from lung cancer. Finally, when control came, it came as the result of the regulatory initiatives of the Secretary of Labor—an agency only tangentially involved with the mining of uranium—and not as a result of the actions of those federal agencies more routinely concerned.
>
> Why did it take so long for government agencies and companies to control the radiation hazard when a technological remedy was available?[4]

Pearson responds to her own question by arguing that several factors played a role in this delay of regulatory and preventive behavior. She argues that the primary factor in this delay was the invisibility of the health threat posed by radiation exposure to miners. She holds that the problem with this invisibility is that it makes public, and thus governmental, recognition of a health problem more difficult.

She supports this hypothesis with a convincing and resourceful study of the relevant variables. First she studies the visibility of health effects of working in a uranium mine. She does this by measuring three variables:

1. The annual incidence of lung cancer deaths among American uranium miners during the period 1950–1970,
2. The annual number of workers' compensation claims filed by uranium miners for lung cancer during the same period, and
3. The number of newspaper articles appearing each year in the popular press about the lung cancer incidence in uranium miners.

Taken together, these three variables give some indication of the visibility of the lung cancer problem among uranium miners. As such, these visibility indices comprise an independent variable: the visibility of radiogenic lung cancers.

Pearson then measures three additional variables:

1. The average number of annual government inspections of each uranium mine from 1950 to 1970,

2. The average radon concentrations in all of the working uranium mines in Colorado during the same period, and

3. The average mining company expenditure for ventilation equipment per ton of mined uranium per year. (This variable is meant to reflect the amount of effort that mining companies put into reducing radon levels in their mines.)

All of these variables are dependent variables that Pearson finds to be related to the independent variable of visibility, as shown in figure 18–1. In her analysis, Pearson finds that the visibility of the problem, as measured by the three variables described above, began to increase in 1957 and reached a peak of visibility in 1966 and 1967. (See figure 18–2). She also found that the incidence of the government inspections began to increase slightly in the late 1950s and peaked in incidence in the late 1960s. (See figure 18–3). In other words, the incidence of government regulatory inspections increased at the same time as, and in response to, the increased visibility of lung cancers among American uranium miners.

In addition, Pearson's statistics strongly suggest that "inspections and sanctions had a dramatic effect on health conditions in the mine."[5] As hazard visibility and mine inspections increased, the amount of money spent by mining companies to reduce radon exposure also increased, and the levels of radon present in the mines fell to more acceptable levels. In summary, Pearson's statistics and historical review suggest the chain of events shown in figure 18–4. As the figure indicates, increased threat visibility leads to increased government regulation, which leads in turn to increased industrial vigilance.

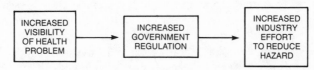

Figure 18–1. Visibility and Uranium Industry Regulation (#1)

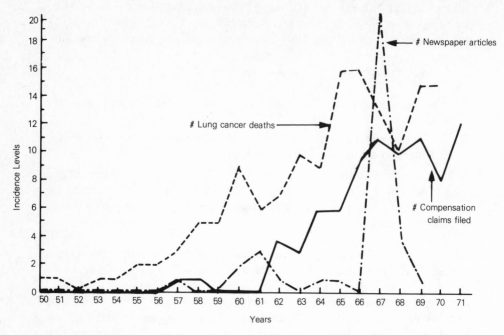

Source: Jessica Pearson, "Hazard Visibility and Occupational Health Problem Solving: The Case of the Uranium Industry," *Journal of Community Health* 6 (1980): 136.

Figure 18–2. Measures of Hazard Visibility

This sequence of events also demonstrates that at least in this particular case there was a period of time during which the involved public and private institutions behaved as though an invisible health threat did not exist in the mines. The Atomic Energy Commission, the government agencies responsible for regulating mining activities, and the mining industry itself refrained from acknowledging the existence of the threat of radiogenic lung cancers to uranium miners until a preponderance of evidence rendered the threat undeniable. The involved institutions denied the existence of this threat even though they were aware of the European studies that had thoroughly documented the problem two decades prior to the creation of the American uranium industry. Despite their awareness of the findings of these studies, they did not take steps to reduce the exposure of American miners to radon, which would have reduced their risk of developing lung cancer.

This phenomenon of the denial of existing invisible health threats by both public and private institutions has not been historically unique to the uranium mining industry. This phenomenon has existed in almost all of the studied accidents involving an exposure to the invisible environmental con-

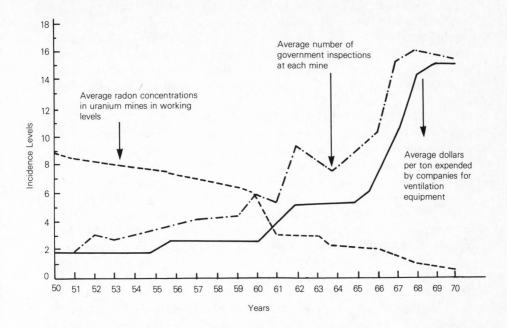

Source: Jessica Pearson, "Hazard Visibility and Occupational Health Problem Solving: The Case of the Uranium Industry," *Journal of Community Health* 6 (1980): 136.

Figure 18–3. Company Expenditures, Government Inspections, and Mine Radiation

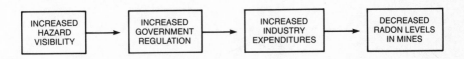

Figure 18–4. Visibility and Uranium Industry Regulation (#2)

taminants.[6] Pearson's case study demonstrates that in the case of uranium mining, the institutional denial of existing invisible threats was permitted because of the environmental and medical invisibility of radiation. The invisibility to the American public of the threat of lung cancer in miners made it possible for industry and government to proceed for two decades as though the threat did not exist.

In this book, we are interested in the institutional denial of invisible threat because of the manner in which these denials exacerbate the untoward psychological effects of the invisible contaminants. Briefly, the institutional denial of invisible threat deepens the uncertainty experienced by exposed individuals because it obscures and obfuscates the real empirical issues that arise for people trying to adapt to an invisible exposure. This institutional denial fosters conditions that encourage the development of the traumatic psychological effects of the invisible contaminants. In addition, if an exposed population senses that an institution is incorrectly denying the existence of an invisible threat, such denials predictably encourage exposed individuals to believe that a serious threat has been or is currently present.[7].

Before giving further documentation of the phenomenon *institutional denial of invisible threat,* I would like to develop a precise definition of the term. Institutions involved in an invisible exposure often contend that the exposure in question posed no threat to the health of exposed individuals. This is an understandable institutional response to an invisible exposure for which the institution may be responsible. The spectrum of conditions under which this institutional position can be taken are as diagrammed in figure 18–5.

Characteristically, two types of institutions are involved with an invisible exposure: (1) the contaminating industry, which is usually a private institution, and (2) the public or governmental institutions responsible for responding to or regulating the contaminating industry. If either of these institutions contends that an invisible health threat does not exist, it is institutional denial of invisible threat if, and only if, that invisible threat actually does exist. (Condition B in the figure.) Thus institutional denial of invisible threat occurs when an institution contends that an invisible health threat does not exist when it actually does exist. The term may also apply to institutional behavior predicated on and expressive of this same position.

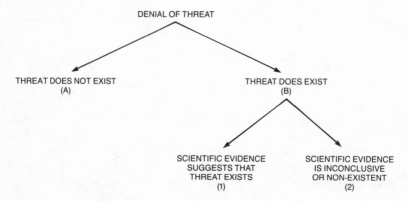

Figure 18–5. Denial of Invisible Threat

One further distinction should be made. Institutional denial of threat can occur under one of two different sets of scientific conditions. It can occur when there is no scientific evidence to support the denial of threat, or when the available scientific evidence actually contradicts the stated denial. In either circumstance, the denying institution is abusing the invisibility of the involved contaminant. They are abusing the invisibility of these contaminants in that they are making empirical statements about the status of an invisible threat that do not adhere to either the data or the usual criteria for making scientific statements. The invisibility of the involved contaminants makes it possible to make such statements without it being apparent that they are inconsistent with existing scientific evidence.

The phenomenon of the institutional denial of invisible threat raises the question of motives. It seems possible that an institution might deny an invisible health threat for any number of reasons. For example, a contaminating industry might deny the existence of an actual threat because it is unaware of the problem. It might deny the existence of the threat because it would cost the institution more money and time than it wishes to expend to change the conditions causing the contamination. Ideological considerations might also lead to an institutional denial of invisible threat. For example, the old Atomic Energy Commission was disbanded and split into two institutions when it was appreciated that the original commission had been charged with carrying out two incompatible missions: the promotion of nuclear energy and the regulation of nuclear energy.[8]

Within the context of our present consideration of the psychological effects of the invisible contaminants, the motives for an institutional denial of invisible threat are both relevant and irrelevant to our understanding of the psychological effects of the invisible contaminants. The issue of institutional motives is irrelevant in that any institutional denial of invisible threat that occurs in the presence of an actual invisible threat will actually increase the uncertainties experienced by individuals attempting to adapt to that threat. Such institutional behavior can only complicate the exposed person's attempts to cope with the effects of that exposure. As an obvious example, people will not be able to protect themselves from an invisible exposure if they do not know and have not been told that it is occurring.

Once again, there is a sense in which the motives of a denying institution are, indeed, relevant to understanding the psychological effects of the invisible environmental contaminants. If an exposed person or population comes to believe that an institution is denying the existence of a past or present invisible threat for self-serving reasons, considerable anger toward that institution will develop in the exposed population. For example, many atomic veterans are very angry at the federal government because they believe that the Veterans Administration and the Defense Nuclear Agency are denying their claims for compensation and medical care for political reasons. They believe that these institutional decisions about their health are predicated on prior policy decisions designed to both save money and protect the government's ability to test and use nuclear weapons.

However, despite the fact that the motives that guide an institution's denial of an invisible threat do matter to the exposed person, and despite the fact that the perception of these motives plays a role in shaping the psychological response to an invisible exposure, there is a larger sense in which institutional motives are irrelevant to the psychological effects of an institutional denial of an invisible threat. No matter what the nature of the institutional motives for denying an invisible threat, the primary effect will always be the same for the concerned person: it will serve to obfuscate his or her attempts to obtain the information needed to adapt to such an exposure. The remainder of this chapter explores the manner in which this occurs and, at the same time, provides further documentation that the institutional denial of invisible threat has not been unique to the uranium mining industry.

Another well-documented example of the institutional denial of invisible threat involves another series of exposures to ionizing radiation. In this instance, the institutional denial of invisible threat involves the behavior of the Department of Defense and the Atomic Energy Commission regarding their atmospheric nuclear weapons testing program at the Nevada Test Site between 1951 and 1962. The United States began the peacetime testing of nuclear weapons immediately after World War II. The first tests were exploded on or near atolls in the South Pacific. However, with the flare up of the Korean War in Asia, it was decided that the South Pacific test site might be lost in a wartime situation and that it would be best to create a test site that would not be vulnerable to enemy attack. As a result, the United States established a nuclear weapons test site within the continental borders of the United States. The site that was chosen is the same site in Nevada where underground nuclear weapons are currently being tested.

One reason that the Nevada location was chosen for the test site was that there is a relatively sparse civilian population living in the areas adjacent to the test site. However, there were and are towns and farms of significant size located within reach of the winds blowing across the Nevada Test Site. Drifting fallout clouds ended up delivering significant and excessive radiation doses to some of those towns and farms.

The consideration, in deciding to perform these tests in remote areas, was to minimize security problems and population exposures to the ionizing radiation released by the bomb tests. This last precaution was taken because it was well known by 1951 that large doses (larger than 100 rads) of radiation could cause acute radiation sickness and that smaller doses could cause a variety of delayed-onset illnesses. The most visible, and thus most widely recognized, of these delayed-onset illnesses were cancers and birth defects.

Ionizing radiation was first discovered in the form of x-rays by Wilhelm Roentgen in 1896. By 1903 it had already been discovered that radiation could cause cancer. By the 1920s it was recognized that ionizing radiation could cause genetic mutations. "By 1950, . . . the concept that genetic alterations [could occur] at any dose of radiation went essentially undisputed among those concerned with radiological protection."[9] Reports of radiogenic cancer continued to emerge throughout this period, and 1949 witnessed the publication of the first Atomic Bomb Casualty Commission paper regarding the appearance of leukemia in a population exposed to fallout from the explosion of an atomic bomb. The Atomic Bomb Casualty Commission was the body established by Japan and the United States to study the health effects of the bombing of Hiroshima and Nagasaki.

It had become evident early on in the history of the clinical and research use of radioactive materials that it was both desirable and necessary for individuals working with these materials to protect themselves from the health effects of radiation. "In 1913, the German Roentgen Society issued the first formal set of guidelines intended for the purpose of reducing exposure to radiation."[10] In 1915 the British Roentgen Society established its own set of guidelines. By 1921, the newly established British X-ray and Radium Protection Committee created a more stringent and comprehensive set of radiation protection rules, which were adopted in 1922 by the American Roentgen Ray Society.

By 1934 the National Council on Radiation Protection of the United States had set a tolerance dose of 0.1 Roentgens per day. The concept of tolerance dose was a pre–World War II protection standard that embodied the notion that below a certain dose radiation would have no harmful biological effects. Shortly after World War II this notion became outdated. Scientists generally came to accept the idea that there is no dose of radiation for which it can be assumed that harmful effects will not occur. In 1954 the National Council on Radiation Protection published a handbook entitled "Permissible Dose From External Sources of Radiation," in which it said that it could no longer assume that there is a radiation threshold dose below which biological damage does not occur.

In keeping with a steadily growing body of knowledge about the biological effects of ionizing radiation,

> standard operating procedures at [the new] national radiation laboratories such as Argonne, Hanford, Oak Ridge and Los Alamos included strict precautions designed to minimize the exposure risk to workers as much as was reasonably practical. . . . [At Oak Ridge] radiation workers were carefully and individually clothed, monitored and decontaminated using both established methods and experimental techniques [as a means of] seeking improvement. They would shower, be checked and shower again to remove any residue. Workers were not permitted to smoke, eat or drink in areas where radioactive contamination was likely to be present. In fact, the laboratory cafeteria was carefully swabbed with absorbent filter paper, which was then counted to detect contamination.[11]

In addition, "the escape of millicuries of radioactive material from Oak Ridge was carefully monitored, with fixed monitoring stations as far as one hundred miles from the laboratory. Research was conducted into aerial monitoring techniques using small planes and specialized instruments. Health physics workers from Oak Ridge would often take instruments into homes in neighboring communities, looking for possible contamination. If radioactivity was found, it was immediately cleaned up."[12]

A completely different approach to radiation monitoring and protection was taken at the Nevada Test Site. The monitoring of off-site radiation exposures resulting from the tests was selective and incomplete. Radiation measurements in the areas of human habitation where contamination occurred and of the residents of those areas were inadequate, in the sense that sufficient measurements were not taken that would have permitted a satisfactory empirical evaluation of whether or not area inhabitants were being exposed to excessive radiation. In his decision in the case of *Allen et al.* vs. *U.S.A.,* Judge Bruce S. Jenkins wrote:

Review of the radiation safety plans and reports as well as more recent analyses of Nevada Test Site monitoring data and the witnesses at trial . . . discloses an astounding fact: at no time during the period 1951 through 1962 did the off-site radiation safety program make any concerted effort to directly monitor and record interval contamination or dosage in off-site residents on a comprehensive person-specific basis. Widespread person-specific monitoring on a random sample basis did not take place until Plumbbob in 1957. Unlike the National Laboratories such as Oak Ridge, where the quantities of material involved were a tiny fraction of those released at [the] Nevada Test Site, no routine urine, fecal or blood samples were taken from residents of local areas exposed to significant, measurable radioactive contamination. Not even in those circumstances where external exposures were estimated to meet or exceed the established safety guidelines, such as in St. George following the Harry Test in May, 1953, did the off-site rad-safe personnel make any effort to check possible internal contamination among residents by direct methods. No thyroid or whole body counters were constructed for use in screening members of the community—especially children—who may have been exposed to more than was permissible even for radiation workers. In fact, in the aftermath of Harry, the monitors decided *not* to take a number of milk samples in order to avoid arousing public concern." [emphasis in the original][13]

Judge Jenkins's assessment is consistent with that of members of the scientific community including Arthur Wolff, who wrote in 1962, as acting chief of the Research Branch, Division of Radiological Health, U.S. Public Health Service, that "no one was looking at the internal exposure picture [at the time of the Harry test] and the tacit assumption has been made that no internal hazards ever existed."[14]

It is worth noting briefly the approach taken by British authorities to a large-scale exposure during the same period. In October 1957 there was a large accident at the plutonium-producing plant at Windscale, England. Approximately 20,000 curies of radioactive iodine-131 were released into the environment. The United Kingdom Atomic Energy Authority initiated an immediate and comprehensive milk-monitoring program in a two-hundred-square-mile area. Milk distribution from a number of neighboring dairy farms was halted for more than a month.

There were other fundamental oversights in the off-site radiation monitoring program at the Nevada Test Site. In general, "the attention of the Nevada Test Site off-site monitoring programs was focused almost exclusively on measurement of external gamma dosage received in the few hours immediately following each detonation." Thus, in addition to measuring only external sources of radiation contamination, Nevada Test Site off-site monitors generally did not measure the levels of external and internal sources of radioactive contamination that were known to persist for long periods after a nuclear bomb explosion.

Despite the fact that the Nevada Test Site radiation monitoring programs did not provide a scientifically complete or accurate picture of the radiation exposures delivered to human beings living within fallout range of the test site, a public information program inaccurately and consistently minimized the radiological dangers posed by the bomb tests to people living within the area. This approach was taken in spite of the "failure of the off-site monitoring programs to gather sufficient information from which to speak with confidence about dose and relative risk to the population exposed to radiation by the nuclear explosions taking place at the test site."[15]

The Atomic Energy Commission established a committee to study the Nevada proving grounds, and the committee issued a report on its findings on February 1, 1954. By then, five series of bomb tests involving thirty-one explosions had been performed at the Nevada Test Site. The committee concluded that "planning did not . . . go very far into the job of assisting safety and of off-setting [public] panic by education, warnings and reports." They went so far as to say that "the need for such actions became obvious . . . [with] the repeated flareup of public concern."

The same Atomic Energy Commission committee found that at least eleven of the thirty-one bomb tests that had been done at that time had "presented a significant hazard as to beta burn and as to whole body gamma exposure, of importance both to domestic animals and to people." Despite the occurrence of these problems, the committee was forced to conclude that with the exception of one occasion, "there had been no specific pre-shot or post-shot warning of probable fallout within the site region, it having been considered necessary on several occasions, but test management having felt that public education and understanding were not sufficiently advanced and that the panic potential was too great."

As a result, test-site authorities mounted a more systematic and visible public education program that centered around the distribution of a pamphlet entitled *Atomic Test Effects in the Nevada Test Site Region*. This booklet came to be regarded as an invaluable tool by test-site authorities: "The most valuable piece of educational material was the little yellow booklet, *Atomic Test Effects in the Nevada Test Site Region*. Thousands of these were distributed through schools, post offices, motels, and by other means."[16]

The pamphlet opens with the statement: "No one inside the Nevada Test Site has been injured as result of the thirty-one test detonations. No one outside the test site in the nearby region of potential exposure has been hurt." The pamphlet also said that "the fallout . . . does not constitute a serious hazard to any living thing outside the test site," and that "no person in the nearby region has been exposed to hazardous amounts of radiation, even from this heavier fallout and no crops or water supplies have been made hazardous to health."[17]

These statements were made even though: (1) adequate environmental and personal monitoring of radiation was not being performed and (2) a previous AEC committee had found that eleven shots had exposed residents and livestock to excessive levels of radiation. It seems fair to conclude that this behavior constitutes an instance of the institutional denial of invisible threat as we defined it earlier.

In addition, during this entire period, the test site was not giving area residents any pretest or posttest information that would enable them to protect themselves from fallout. In general, test-site personnel attempted to keep such warnings to an absolute minimum. They effected this policy by unilaterally raising the level of radiation to which the public could be exposed—with or without notification. This approach was outlined in a 1952 Nevada Test Site document as follows:

> In considering the levels of radiation to which the general public might permissibly be exposed, we have tried to keep in mind the somewhat delicate public relations aspect of the affair. . . . It is felt that [exposure] figures must be used as general guides but that no drastic action which might disturb the public should be taken unless it is clearly felt that such action is essential to protect local residents from almost certain damage. It is assumed that any member of the general public may receive external exposure up to twenty-five rads without danger. . . . For areas where exposure above fifty rads may occur, consideration must of necessity be given to evacuating personnel, but such a step would not be taken unless it is firmly regarded as essential.[18]

This policy became Nevada Test Site operating procedure even though the maximal permissible dose for employees in the nuclear industry was 3.9 rads per three months. This figure had been established by the National Council on Radiation Protection. The approach of test-site personnel to civilian exposures seems to have been one of ongoing institutional denial of invisible threat.

The Nevada Test Site's approach to radiation monitoring and public information can be best understood as a program to prevent the occurrence of any of the symptoms of acute radiation sickness among the residents of the test-site area. Judge Jenkins found that:[19]

1. "The off-site monitoring activities at Nevada Test Site between 1951 and 1962 were overwhelmingly geared toward assessment of the first, acute phase of fallout hazard," and

2. There was a "consistent pattern of risk assessment that focuse(d) almost entirely on acute exposure rates, risks and biological consequences."

In other words, the Nevada Test Site focused on preventing radiation exposures that would cause the immediate and thus visible appearance of symptoms. Once again, radiation exposure can cause two basic classes of illness: (1) acute radiation sickness, which appears within hours or days of a large (greater than 75 rads) exposure and (2) the various forms of delayed radiation illness that will appear three to thirty-five years after the occurrence of smaller exposures. The Nevada Test Site safety and public education program appears to have been concerned with the prevention of only acute radiation sickness—those forms of radiation illness that would be visible at the time of the bomb tests. The Nevada Test Site safety program was not designed to prevent the occurrence of the invisible or delayed-onset forms of radiation illness.

In summary, Judge Jenkins found that

> the information provided to persons living in the off-site area surrounding the Nevada Test Site was woefully deficient in at least three respects: public · education relating to the nature and extent of hazards—particularly the long-term risks associated with radiation exposure—was not adequate to inform off-site residents of the foreseeable risks arising from exposure to fallout in that area; nor was sufficient information provided to educate people as to the precautionary measures that they could take to protect themselves, to minimize the degree of fallout contamination. . . . Finally, warnings given at crucial times failed to provide enough information soon enough to be useful and effective.[20]

This state of affairs endured for many years, creating an ongoing situation in which area residents knew that they were being exposed to radiation without understanding how to adapt to or protect themselves from that fallout. The government did not supply test-area residents with the information that they would have needed to successfully adapt to the threats posed to their health by the fallout. It was actually possible for the involved government institutions to portray, for a time, the situation as one in which significant threats did not exist. It was possible to do this because of the environmental and medical invisibility of radiation.

As we have seen, the process of adapting to a threat requires the accumulation and analysis of information about that threat. We have also seen that lack of information about a threat can change the process of adaptation in predictable ways and even cause the development of untoward psychological effects such as: (1) profound fear and uncertainty, (2) hypervigilance, (3) changed images of self and world mediated by nonempirical belief systems about the threat, and (4) traumatic neuroses. In recognition of this dynamic, it seems safe to conclude that the institutional denial of threat exacerbates, or even creates, situations in which the adverse psychological effects of an invisible contamination are likely to develop. By withholding information and presenting inaccurate information, the Nevada Test Site personnel made it virtually impossible for test-site area residents to successfully adapt to their invisible exposures to radiation.

The phenomenon of the institutional denial of invisible threat is not unique to contaminations involving radiation. These institutional denials have also occurred in response to exposures involving the toxic chemicals. Institutional denial of invisible threat has been documented in the cooking oil contamination in western Japan,[21] the dioxin contamination in Italy,[22] the livestock feed contamination in Michigan,[23] the occupational exposures to toxic chemicals,[24] and the Love Canal contamination.[25]

At the beginning of the Love Canal disaster, the New York State Department of Health concluded as a result of both environmental studies and preliminary medical studies that two segments of the Love Canal neighborhood were not safe for human habitation. As a result, the state bought the houses located in those two areas—rings I and II—thus making it possible for area residents to move and live elsewhere. The state did not purchase homes in the one remaining segment of the Love Canal neighborhood—ring III. As recounted in chapter 7, the state later: (1) announced that it was going to perform additional studies of the health effects of the canal, (2) told ring III residents that the state would not purchase ring III homes because it was safe to live in that part of the Love Canal neighborhood, and (3) appealed to the federal government for funds with which to purchase ring III housing.[26] It would be fair to say that during this period the state began to take a rather leisurely approach to doing additional health studies of ring III residents.

There is a contradiction here: the state was telling ring III residents that it was safe to live in ring III in the absence of data that empirically indicated its safety. If anything, the existing health studies of ring III residents suggested that it was actually dangerous to live in ring III. A state health department study had already found increased rates of negative birth outcomes in the drainage areas of ring III, and an Environmental Protection Agency pilot study had found chromosomal damage among ring III residents. The effects of this institutional denial of invisible threat were predictable.

As time passed, ring III residents became more and more convinced that they were living in a dangerous situation. Several events occurred that both encouraged and confirmed their belief (see page 46 of chapter 7 for a listing of these events). They found themselves living in a situation that they regarded as dangerous, but from which they could not escape. Their ability to escape was financially contingent upon institutional confirmation of an invisible threat, but the involved institutions continued to claim that the situation was safe.

The magnitude of the psychological impact of this institutional denial of invisible threat reached such obvious proportions that when the federal government did eventually give the state of New York the financial assistance it needed to purchase ring III housing, it did so on the grounds that there was a "mental health emergency" at Love Canal. The funding was not given to New York on the grounds that either the New York State Department of Health or the Environmental Protection Agency had determined that a physical health hazard was present in ring III of the Love Canal neighborhood.

During the period of frozen adaptation that surrounded the contemplated purchase of ring III housing, several things seem to have happened: (1) the residents of ring III came to believe that their health was threatened by the Love Canal and they developed belief systems that embodied the notion, (2) they became fearful and uncertain about the ongoing and cumulative health impacts of living in proximity to the canal, and (3) they partially delegated the important task of monitoring the health effects of the canal to the governmental institutions that were doing scientific studies of the canal. When the government proved to be less than responsible in carrying out its duties, the community panicked—the most severe form of hypervigilance.

The sequence of events at Love Canal is shown in figure 18–6.

In this situation, institutional denial of invisible threat seems to have played a definite role in precipitating the fear, uncertainty, and hypervigilance of ring III residents. In this instance, public policy thwarted the ability of area residents to adapt to an invisible threat. The result was an avoidable "mental health emergency" that required an evacuation anyway.

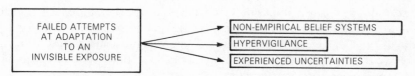

Figure 18–6. Failed Attempts at Adaptation

There are often genuine considerations that lead institutions to minimize or deny the presence of an invisible threat. As the Atomic Energy Commission stated in its 1954 evaluation of Nevada Test Site management, management personnel felt that giving the public warning of potential or actual fallout dangers was inadvisable because "the panic potential was too great."[27] However, as the above examples clearly and ironically illustrate, it is the very withholding of information itself that causes panic and psychological trauma in an exposed community. The implications of these findings for public policy seem clear. We have looked at three case studies of the psychosocial consequences of situations in which institutions have attempted to minimize information concerning the danger of an invisible exposure: downwind Utah, the atomic veterans, and Love Canal. In all three situations, the denial strategy did not prevent the occurrence of hypervigilant responses to a contamination. The residents of southwestern Utah became demonstrably concerned about the fallout clouds passing over their heads.[28] The atomic veterans eventually became preoccupied with their health.[29] The residents of Love Canal panicked several times in the course of the protracted disaster situation created by the canal.[30]

There is, on the other hand, evidence to suggest that information about an invisible contamination will cause an exposed population to panic and become hypervigilant. There was panic at Three Mile Island after the governor's evacuation announcement. There was certainly panic present in the methyl alcohol poisoning in Atlanta; over half of the people who reported to the hospital for treatment did not have any of the symptoms of methyl alcohol poisoning. There was evident panic in the PCB contamination in Japan; something on the order of 10 percent of the people reporting to public health centers for treatment actually had the symptoms of PCB contamination.

It appears, then, that panic and hypervigilance will develop in consequence of an invisible exposure regardless of which approach is taken. Hypervigilance will occur if notification of contamination occurs at the time of an exposure, and it will occur if notification is given at a later date—as in the case of an institutional denial of invisible threat. Present data indicate that panic and hypervigilance are an inevitable part of the response to an invisible contamination. Thus it makes no sense to deny, as a matter of policy, the presence or effects of an invisible contaminant as a means of preventing hypervigilance and panic. Portraying an invisible threat as being safe does not accomplish its declared end of preventing panic in an exposed population. At best, it delays the appearance of hypervigilance. However, in so doing, such policy runs the risk of entrenching the exposed person or persons in a life pattern of hypervigilance. As we have seen, hypervigilance can actually become, over a period of protracted concern and failed adaptation, a way of life for the exposed person.[31]

Thus the denial or minimization of invisible threat appears to be bad policy for a number of reasons:

1. It does not prevent the hypervigilance and panic it is designed to prevent.
2. It encourages the development of psychological trauma in some members of the exposed population.
3. It places people at the additional risk of developing somatic illness as a result of an invisible contamination.

It seems fair to conclude, then, that even though both acknowledgment and denial of an invisible threat produce panic and hypervigilance in an exposed population, it is far better for institutions to inform a population of the dangers they face. This approach avoids the problems described above and gives exposed individuals the best chance of making a successful and empirically informed adaptation to an invisible exposure.

Finally, I suspect that panic and hypervigilance would be reduced to a minimum if an exposed person or population were told that:

1. They were in the process of being exposed to an invisible contaminant or that they were already at increased risk of developing contaminant-caused disease,
2. It is difficult to know with certainty how to best adapt to an exposure to an invisible contaminant because of its environmental and medical invisibility, but
3. The involved institutions are aware of that difficulty and will do their best to help the exposed population to prevent and minimize exposure, and monitor the health effects of that exposure.

The basic thrust of public policy in the instance of an invisible exposure should always be to assist the exposed population in the tasks of adapting to the threats posed by that exposure.

19
Epilogue:
A Nation of Hypochondriacs

Given that it is possible for people who have been accidentally exposed to an invisible environmental contaminant to develop various traumatic consequences of those exposures, what does this mean for the rest of us? Are these psychological traumata a harbinger of larger changes to come in our society? Or are they an isolated phenomenon that happens only to those people who have been through a major accidental exposure to an invisible contaminant? Will there be more and more of us who become preoccupied with our health and the dangers of the contaminants in our environment as pollution continues to be a part of our lives? Will the growing number of people who live near or work in contaminant-producing facilities experience the same problems as the people who have been studied in this book? Or is this a more limited phenomenon?

Empirical answers to these questions are not available at this time. We do not know enough about the psychosocial effects of the invisible environmental contaminants to make any predictions about the future. But I do think that it is prudent to ask these questions now, and within that context, I would like to make a few brief observations.

There is growing concern in this country with the dangers of environmental contamination. Sometimes it seems as if we are living in a world in which almost everything is being indicted as a carcinogen. The media are full of scientific reports of the carcinogenic properties of one substance or another. The persistent fascination of the media with carcinogenicity can only be a reflection of the interest that their audience has in knowing about these matters.

There is also a large environmentalist movement. The existence and national political impact of this movement suggest that there are a considerable number of people in this country who have become concerned about both the health effects and the ecological effects of the environmental contaminants. The size of this movement is an indication of the number of people who have begun the historical task of worrying about the effects of environmental pollution. By historical, I mean that it is now becoming a historical fact that two centuries after the inception of the industrial age, noticeable segments of modern society are becoming concerned about the effects of industrial pollution.

Douglas and Wildavsky have made some very interesting observations about the environmentalist movement. They contend, in *Culture and Risk,* that this movement can be better understood as a cultural phenomenon than as a group of people genuinely concerned with the objective dangers of the environmental contaminants.[1] They see the environmentalist concern with contamination as part of that recognizable cultural, or sectarian, dynamic in which a social group defines itself and holds itself apart from other groups through the creation òf pollution beliefs. The ancient Jews distinguished themselves from other peoples by not eating the meat of pigs. Amish prohibitions against participating in modern life set the Amish apart. Douglas and Wildavsky argue that the environmentalist movement is a sectarian group with a distinctive world view that sees environmental contaminants as polluting because they are part of a way of life—the centrist corporate industrial life of the United States—different from the environmentalists' own.

There is much that is anthropologically correct in this analysis, but one is forced to conclude that this analysis is incomplete. It seems only obvious that genuinely dangerous phenomena can and do become the object of pollution belief and practice. The incorporation by a social group of a real danger with which it lives into a pollution belief dynamic does not mean that the threat in question is not genuine. The industrial contaminants that are regarded as pollutants by those with environmental concerns do actually cause cancer and other illnesses. It would be a mistake to regard these contaminants as safe just because they are part of a pollution dynamic. Unlike the cultural categories that underly pollution beliefs, a culturally defined pollutant can also be a genuine threat to a people's health and welfare.

This brings us back to the question of whether industrial pollution is changing the collective realities with which we envision our world. Will it change us, or many of us, into a nation of people preoccupied with our health and the potential hostility of our environment? Is concern about environmental contaminants the sole province of the environmentalists, or is it a concern that belongs to broader segments of the American public? Will these concerns become entrenched in our lives in the same manner in which they have become entrenched in the lives of the atomic veterans? Will we become a nation of so-called hypochondriacs?

In asking these questions, I am not suggesting that this is necessarily the case. But I think it would have sounded equally preposterous, two centuries ago, to have raised the question of whether Lake Erie would almost die at the end of the twentieth century, or to have asked, even fifty years ago, whether human beings might some day dismantle the ozone layer of the atmosphere.

I think it is important, given the findings of this book, to ask how environmental pollution is changing us as a people. If we ask these questions now, perhaps we will find that there is nothing to concern us, that the psychological effects of the invisible environmental contaminants as documented in this book are something that happens only to those people who have experienced significant exposures. If this is the case, then all that need be done is to take steps to minimize the occurrence of the accidental exposures and to learn to deal with them in an effective manner when they do occur. On the other hand, if we observe by asking these questions now that the psychosocial effects of the invisible contaminants are becoming a presence in the everyday life of the country, we would then be in a position to reverse this process.

While we are asking these questions, we can note that all evidence indicates that adapting to an invisible exposure is a toxic process. It is a process that can severely traumatize the exposed persons and change their lives for the worse. Under these circumstances, it seems only just that we do everything we can, as a society, to prevent the occurrence of these exposures and to assure, once an accident has happened, that all self-interest be dropped in order to help the exposed people adapt to a most difficult and uncertain situation.

Notes

Chapter 1

1. Geoffrey Marks, *The Medieval Plague* (Garden City, N.Y.: Doubleday, 1971); Anna M. Campbell, *The Black Death and Learning* (New York: Columbia University Press, 1931).

2. Robert J. Lifton, *Death in Life* (New York: Random House, 1967).

3. Henry M. Vyner, "The Psychological Effects of Ionizing Radiation," *Culture, Medicine and Psychiatry* 7 (1983): 241–63.

4. Adeline G. Levine, *Love Canal: Science, Politics and People* (Lexington, Mass.: Lexington Books, 1982); Martha R. Fowlkes and P.Y. Miller, "Love Canal: The Social Construction of Disaster" (Submitted to the Federal Emergency Management Agency, October 1982).

5. Michael R. Reich, "Toxic Politics: A Comparative Study of Public and Private Responses to Chemical Disasters in the United States, Italy and Japan" (Ph.D. dissertation, Yale University, 1982).

6. Ibid.

7. Carroll M. Brodsky, "Psychological Factors Contributing to Somatoform Diseases Attributed to the Workplace," *Journal of Occupational Medicine* 25, no. 6 (1983): 459–464; Dorothy Nelkin and Michael Brown, *Workers at Risk* (Chicago: University of Chicago Press, 1984).

8. Peter Houts et al., "Health Related Behavioral Impact of the Three Mile Island Incident," parts I, II, III (Submitted to the Three Mile Island Advisory Panel on Health Research Studies of the Pennsylvania Department of Health, 1981); Field Research Corporation, *Public Opinion in Pennsylvania Toward the Accident at Three Mile Island and Its Aftermath* (San Francisco: Field Research Corporation, 1980); Henry M. Vyner, "Belief Systems in the Three Mile Island Area Population" (Presented at the Three Mile Island Public Health Fund's Forum on the Health Effects of Ionizing Radiation, Harrisburg, Penn., March 30, 1983).

9. Reich, "Toxic Politics."

10. Evelyn Bromet et al., "Preliminary Report on the Mental Health of the Three Mile Island Residents" (Submitted to the Department of Health and Human Services, National Institute of Mental Health, Disaster Assistance and Emergency Mental Health Section, May 1981); Andrew Baum et al., "Chronic and Acute Stress Associated With the Three Mile Island Accident and Decontamination: Preliminary

Findings of a Longitudinal Study" (Submitted to the Nuclear Regulatory Commission, July 1981).

Chapter 2

1. Geoffrey Marks, *The Medieval Plague* (Garden City, N.Y.: Doubleday, 1971).
2. Ibid.
3. Ibid.
4. F.P. Wilson, *The Plague in Shakespeare's London* (Oxford: Clarendon Press, 1927).
5. Anna M. Campbell, *The Black Death and Learning* (New York: Columbia University Press, 1931), 37.
6. Ibid., 41.
7. Ibid.
8. Ibid.
9. Ibid.
10. Marks, *Medieval Plague.*
11. Ibid.

Chapter 3

1. Adeline G. Levine, "The Psychosocial Impact of Toxic Chemical Waste Dumps," *Environmental Health Perspectives* 48 (1983): 15–17.
2. Adeline G. Levine, "Love Canal: Scientific Controversy and Policy Dilemma" (Presented at the Institute of Environmental Health, April 1983), 10.
3. Michael R. Reich, "Toxic Politics: A Comparative Study of Public and Private Responses to Chemical Disasters in the United States, Italy and Japan" (Ph.D. dissertation, Yale University, 1982).
4. Ibid., 142.

Chapter 4

1. F.P. Wilson, *The Plague in Shakespeare's London* (Oxford: Clarendon Press, 1927).
2. Geoffrey Marks, *The Medieval Plague* (Garden City, N.Y.: Doubleday, 1971).
3. Richard S. Lazarus, *Psychological Stress and the Coping Process* (New York: McGraw Hill, 1966), 117.
4. Martha R. Fowlkes and P.Y. Miller, "Love Canal: The Social Construction of Disaster" (Submitted to the Federal Emergency Management Agency, October 1982), 44–45.
5. Andrew Baum et al., "Chronic and Acute Stress Associated With the Three Mile Island Accident and Decontamination: Preliminary Findings of a Longitudinal Study" (Submitted to the Nuclear Regulatory Commission, July 1981).

6. Henry M. Vyner, "The Psychological Effects of Ionizing Radiation," *Culture, Medicine and Psychiatry* 7 (1983): 241–63.

7. Michael R. Reich, "Toxic Politics: A Comparative Study of Public and Private Responses to Chemical Disasters in the United States, Italy and Japan" (Ph.D. dissertation, Yale University, 1982).

8. Ibid.

9. Ibid.

10. J.W. Powell, "A Poison Liquor Episode in Atlanta, Georgia" (Presented at Conference on Field Studies on Reactions to Disasters, National Opinion Research Center, 1953).

11. Fowlkes and Miller, "Love Canal."

12. Adeline G. Levine, *Love Canal: Science, Politics and People* (Lexington, Mass.: Lexington Books, 1982).

13. Vyner, "Ionizing Radiation."

14. Henry M. Vyner, "Belief Systems in the Three Mile Island Area Population" (Presented at the Three Mile Island Public Health Fund's Forum on the Health Effects of Ionizing Radiation, Harrisburg, Penn., March 30, 1983).

15. Francis L.K. Hsu, "A Cholera Epidemic in a Chinese Town," in *Health, Culture and Community,* ed. B.D. Paul (New York: Russell Sage Foundation, 1955), 135–54.

16. John Cassell, "A Comprehensive Health Program Among South African Zulus," in *Health, Culture and Community,* ed. B.D. Paul (New York: Russell Sage Foundation, 1955), 15–54.

17. Ibid.

Chapter 5

1. C.B. Flynn, "Three Mile Island Telephone Survey" (Submitted to the Nuclear Regulatory Commission, September 1979), 14.

2. Henry M. Vyner, "The Psychosocial Effects of the Invisible Environmental Contaminants" (Presented to the Three Mile Island Public Health Fund's Workshop on the Psychosocial Effects of the Invisible Environmental Contaminants, June 1984).

3. Michael R. Reich, "Toxic Politics: A Comparative Study of Public and Private Responses to Chemical Disasters in the United States, Italy and Japan" (Ph.D. dissertation, Yale University, 1982), 149.

4. I.L. Janis, "Psychological Effects of Warning," in *Man and Society in Disaster,* eds. G.W. Baker and D.W. Chapman (New York: Basic Books, 1962), 55–92.

5. Flynn, "Three Mile Island"; Peter Houts et al., "Health Related Behavioral Impact of the Three Mile Island Incident," part I (Submitted to the Three Mile Island Advisory Panel on Health Research Studies of the Pennsylvania Department of Health, 1981), 14.

6. Henry M. Vyner, "The Psychological Effects of Ionizing Radiation," *Culture, Medicine and Psychiatry* 7 (1983): 241–63.

7. Reich, "Toxic Politics."

8. Adeline G. Levine, *Love Canal: Science, Politics and People* (Lexington, Mass.: Lexington Books, 1982); Martha R. Fowlkes and P.Y. Miller, "Love Canal:

The Social Construction of Disaster" (Submitted to the Federal Emergency Management Agency, October 1982).

9. Henry M. Vyner, unpublished interview with an atomic veteran, October 1980.

Chapter 6

1. Michael R. Reich, "Toxic Politics: A Comparative Study of Public and Private Responses to Chemical Disasters in the United States, Italy and Japan" (Ph.D. dissertation, Yale University, 1982), 26.
2. Ibid., 34.
3. Ibid., 42.
4. Ibid., 48.
5. Ibid., 51.
6. Ibid., 50.
7. Ibid., 50.
8. Ibid., 54–55.
9. Ibid., 39.
10. Ibid., 40.
11. Ibid., 58.
12. Ibid., 59.

Chapter 7

1. Adeline G. Levine, *Love Canal: Science, Politics and People* (Lexington, Mass.: Lexington Books, 1982), 14.
2. Ibid., 22.
3. Ibid., 28.
4. Martha R. Fowlkes and P.Y. Miller, "Love Canal: The Social Construction of Disaster" (Submitted to the Federal Emergency Management Agency, October 1982), 14.
5. Levine, *Love Canal,* 83.
6. Fowlkes and Miller, "Love Canal," 17; Levine, *Love Canal,* 129.
7. Levine, *Love Canal,* 120.
8. Fowlkes and Miller, "Love Canal," 11–12.
9. Levine, *Love Canal,* 101.
10. Ibid., 144.
11. Adeline G. Levine, "Psychosocial Effects of Toxic Waste Dumps," *Environmental Health Perspectives* 48 (1983): 17.
12. Fowlkes and Miller, "Love Canal," 20.

Chapter 9

1. Michael R. Reich, "Toxic Politics: A Comparative Study of Public and Private Responses to Chemical Disasters in the United States, Italy and Japan" (Ph. D. dissertation, Yale University, 1982), 213–14.

2. Martha R. Fowlkes and P.Y. Miller, "Love Canal: The Social Construction of Disaster" (Submitted to the Federal Emergency Management Agency, October 1982), 44.

3. Adeline G. Levine, *Love Canal: Science, Politics and People* (Lexington, Mass.: Lexington Books, 1982), 7–8.

4. Henry M. Vyner, "The Psychological Effects of Ionizing Radiation," *Culture, Medicine and Psychiatry* 7 (1983): 241–63.

5. Andrew Baum et al., "Chronic and Acute Stress Associated With the Three Mile Island Accident and Decontamination: Preliminary Findings of a Longitudinal Study" (Submitted to the Nuclear Regulatory Commission, July 1981).

6. K. Lang and G. Lang, *Collective Dynamics* (New York: Crowell, 1961), 71.

7. Henry M. Vyner, "Psychological Effects," 248.

8. Ibid.

9. B.B. Hudson, "Anxiety in Response to the Unfamiliar," *Journal of Social Issues* 10 (1954): 53–60.

10. Henry M. Vyner, Unpublished interviews from pilot study for Three Mile Island survey, November 1981.

11. Defense Nuclear Agency, *Nuclear Test Personnel Review* (Washington, D.C.: Department of Defense, 1981).

12. Reich, "Toxic Politics."

13. Dorothy Nelkin and M.R. Brown. *Workers at Risk* (Chicago: University of Chicago Press, 1984), 30.

14. Vyner, "Psychological Effects."

15. Fowlkes and Miller, "Love Canal."

16. C.M. Brodsky, "Psychological Factors Contributing to Somatoform Diseases, Attributed to the Workplace," *Journal of Occupational Medicine* 25, no. 6 (1983): 459–64.

17. Reich, "Toxic Politics."

Chapter 10

1. K.N. Prasad, *CRC Handbook of Radiobiology* (Boca Raton, Fla.: CRC Press, 1984), 98.

2. John W. Gofman, *Radiation and Human Health* (San Francisco: Sierra Club Books, 1981), 637.

3. Ibid., 52.

4. W.M. Wintrobe et al., eds., *Harrison's Principles of Internal Medicine* (New York: McGraw-Hill, 1970).

5. V.N. Strel'Tsova, "General Aspects of the Remote Aftereffects of Radiation Damage and Means for Studying Them," in *Remote Aftereffects of Radiation,* ed. by Yu. I. Moskalev, trans. National Technical Information Service (Moscow: Atomizdat, 1971), 5–38.

6. Richard S. Lazarus, *Psychological Stress and the Coping Process* (New York: McGraw-Hill, 1966); Richard S. Lazarus and R. Launier, "Stress Related Transactions Between Person and Environment," in *Perspectives in Interactional Psychology,* ed. by L.A. Pervin and M. Lewis (New York: Plenum Press, 1981), 287–327; Richard S. Lazarus, "The Stress and Coping Paradigm," in *Models Clin-*

Richard S. Lazarus, "The Stress and Coping Paradigm," in *Models for Clinical Psychopathology,* ed. by C. Eisdorfer et al. (New York: Spectrum, 1981), 177–214.

7. Lazarus, *Psychological Stress,* 25.

8. Ibid., 30.

9. Ibid., 25.

10. Hans Selye, *The Stress of Life* (New York: McGraw-Hill, 1956).

11. Lazarus, "Stress and Coping Paradigm," 178.

12. Ibid., 178.

13. Richard S. Lazarus et al., "Toward a Cognitive Theory of Emotions," in *Feelings and Emotions,* ed. by M. Arnold (New York: Academic Press, 1970), 207–32.

14. Lazarus, *Psychological Stress,* 5.

15. Ibid; J.W. Mason, "A Historical View of the Stress Field," *Journal of Human Stress* 1 (1975): 22–36.

16. Lazarus, *Psychological Stress,* 27.

17. Ibid., 17.

18. Ibid., 7–8.

19. Lazarus, "Stress and Coping Paradigm," 178.

20. Lazarus and Launier, "Stress Related Transactions," 298.

21. Ibid., 302.

22. Lazarus, "Stress and Coping Paradigm," 192.

23. Lazarus, *Psychological Stress.*

24. Lazarus and Launier, "Stress Related Transactions," 306.

25. Lazarus, "Stress and Coping Paradigm," 195.

26. Lazarus and Launier, "Stress Related Transactions," 306.

27. Ibid., 296.

28. Ibid., 311.

29. Lazarus, "Stress and Coping Paradigm"; David Mechanic, *Students Under Stress* (New York: The Free Press, 1962).

30. Irving L. Janis and L. Mann, *Decision Making* (New York: The Free Press, 1977).

31. David A. Hamburg and J.E. Adams, "A Perspective on Coping: Seeking and Utilizing Information in Major Transitions," *Archives of General Psychiatry, 1967* 17 (1967): 277–84.

32. Susan Folkman et al., "Cognitive Processes as Mediators of Stress and Coping," in *Human Stress and Cognition: An Information Processing Approach,* ed. by V. Hamilton and D.M. Warburton: (Chichester, England: Wiley, 1979), 265–98.

33. Lazarus, "The Stress and Coping Paradigm," 200.

34. Irving L. Janis, *Psychological Stress: Psychoanalytic and Behavioral Studies of Surgical Patients* (New York: Wiley, 1958); Richard S. Lazarus, "Emotions and Perceptions: Conceptual and Empirical Relations," *Nebraska Symposium on Motivation,* ed. by W.J. Arnold (Lincoln: University of Nebraska Press, 1968).

35. Irving L. Janis, "Psychological Effects of Warnings," in *Man and Society in Disaster,* ed. by G.W. Baker and D.W. Chapman (New York: Basic Books, 1962), 55–92; Janis and Mann, *Decision Making*; Henry M. Vyner, "The Psychological Effects of Ionizing Radiation," *Culture, Medicine and Psychiatry* 7 (1983): 241–63; Martha R. Fowlkes and P.Y. Miller, "Love Canal: The Social Construction of Disaster" (Submitted to the Federal Emergency Management Agency, October 1982);

Michael R. Reich, "Toxic Politics: A Comparative Study of Public and Private Responses to Chemical Disasters in the United States, Italy and Japan" (Ph.D. dissertation, Yale University, 1982); Adeline G. Levine, *Love Canal: Science, Politics and People* (Lexington, Mass.: Lexington Books, 1982).

36. Lazarus, "Stress and Coping Paradigm"; Janis, "Psychological Effects"; Janis and Mann, *Decision Making.*

37. Janis and Mann, *Decision Making.*

38. Ibid.

39. J.W. Powell, "A Poison Liquor Episode in Atlanta, Georgia" (Presented to Conference of Field Studies on Reactions to Disasters, National Opinion Research Center, Chicago, 1953).

40. C. Fritz and E. Marks, "The NORC Studies of Human Behavior in Disaster," *Journal of Social Issues* 10 (1954): 26–41; Janis, 1962, "Psychological Effects."

41. Henry M. Vyner, "The Psychosocial Effects of the Invisible Environmental Contaminants" (Presented at the Three Mile Island Public Health Fund's Workshop on the Psychosocial Effects of the Invisible Environmental Contaminants, June 1984).

42. Reich, "Toxic Politics"; Levine, *Love Canal*; C.M. Brodsky, "Psychological Factors Contributing to Somatoform Diseases Attributed to the Workplace," *Journal of Occupational Medicine* 25, no. 6 (1983): 459–64; Fowlkes and Miller, "Love Canal."

43. Lazarus, *Psychological Stress;* George Mandler, "Thought Processes, Consciousness and Stress," in *Human Stress and Cognition,* ed. by V. Hamilton and D.M. Warburton (Chichester, England: Wiley, 1979); V. Hamilton and D.M. Warburton, eds. *Human Stress and Cognition: An Information Processing Approach* (Chichester, England: Wiley, 1979); B. Shalit, "The Perception of Threat by a Noxious Gas Accident and the Reported Coping Style" (In press).

44. Shalit, "Perception of Threat."

45. Folkman, "Cognitive Processes," 276.

46. Lazarus and Launier, "Stress Related Transactions"; R.S. Lazarus et al., "A Laboratory Study of Psychological Stress Produced by a Motion Picture Film," *Psychological Monographs* 76 (1962): 34.

Chapter 11

1. Susan Sontag, *Illness as Metaphor* (New York: Vintage Books, 1979).

2. C.M. Brodsky, "Psychological Factors Contributing to Somatoform Diseases Attributed to the Workplace," *Journal of Occupational Medicine* 25, no. 6 (1983): 459–64.

3. Field Research Corporation, *Public Opinion in Pennsylvania Toward the Accident at Three Mile Island and Its Aftermath* (San Francisco: Field Research Corporation, 1980); Peter Houts et al., "Health Related Behavioral Impact of the Three Mile Island Nuclear Incident," part I (Submitted to the Three Mile Island Advisory Panel on Health Research Studies of the Pennsylvania Department of Health, 1981).

4. Adeline Levine, *Love Canal: Science, Politics and People* (Lexington, Mass.: Lexington Books, 1982); Martha R. Fowlkes and P.Y. Miller, "Love Canal: The

Social Construction of Disaster" (Submitted to the Federal Emergency Management Agency, October 1982).

5. Henry M. Vyner, "The Psychological Effects of Ionizing Radiation," *Culture, Medicine and Psychiatry* 7 (1983): 241–63.

6. Brodsky, "Psychological Factors."

7. Henry M. Vyner, "Belief Systems in the Three Mile Island Area Population" (Presented at the Three Mile Island Public Health Fund's Forum on the Health Effects of Ionizing Radiation, Harrisburg, Penn., March 1980).

8. Vyner, "Psychological Effects of Radiation," 248–49.

9. Vyner, "Psychological Effects of Radiation"; Fowlkes and Miller, "Love Canal"; Levine, *Love Canal;* Brodsky, "Psychological Factors."

10. Vyner, "Belief Systems"; Fowlkes and Miller, "Love Canal."

11. Vyner, "Belief Systems"; Fowlkes and Miller, "Love Canal."

12. Fowlkes and Miller, "Love Canal," 95.

13. Ibid.

14. Levine, *Love Canal.*

15. Houts, "Health Related Behavioral Impact"; Robert Del Tredici, *The People of Three Mile Island* (San Francisco: Sierra Club Books, 1983); Robert Leppzer, *Voices From Three Mile Island* (Trumansburg, N.Y.: The Crossing Press, 1982); H. Wasserman and N. Solomon, *Killing Our Own* (New York: Dell, 1982); Houts, "Health Related Behavioral Impact."

16. Ibid.

17. Field Research Corporation, *Public Opinion.*

18. Vyner, "Belief Systems."

19. Ibid.

20. Brodsky, "Psychological Factors," 460.

21. Vyner, "The Psychological Effects of Radiation."

22. Fowlkes and Miller, "Love Canal."

23. Houts, "Health Related Behavioral Impact"; Vyner, "Belief Systems"; Henry M. Vyner, "Post-Exposure Health Care for Patients Exposed to Radiation and the Other Invisible Environmental Contaminants," *Social Science and Medicine* (in press).

24. Levine, *Love Canal;* Fowlkes and Miller, "Love Canal."

25. Vyner, "Belief Systems"; Vyner, "Post-Exposure Health Care"; Houts, "Health Related Behavioral Impact."

26. Vyner, "Psychological Effects of Radiation."

27. Brodsky, "Psychological Factors."

28. Richard S. Lazarus, *Psychological Stress and the Coping Process* (New York: McGraw-Hill, 1966), 117–18.

29. Ibid., 117.

30. Lazarus, *Psychological Stress;* S.B. Withey, "Reaction to Uncertain Threat," in *Man and Society in Disaster,* ed. by G.W. Baker and D.W. Chapman (New York: Basic Books, 1962), 93–123.

31. J.R. Averill, "Personality Control Over Aversive Stimuli and Its Relation to Stress," *Psychological Bulletin* 80 (1973): 286–303; G. Ball and R. Vogler, "Uncertain Pain and the Pain of Uncertainty," *Perceptual Motor Skills* 33 (1971): 1195–1203; A.S. Dibner, "Ambiguity and Anxiety," *Journal of Abnormal and Social Psychology* 56 (1958): 165–74; E. Frenkel-Brunswick, "Intolerance of Ambiguity as an Emotional and Perceptual Variable," *Journal of Personality* 18 (1949): 108–43.

32. Ball and Vogler, "Uncertain Pain."

33. Averill, "Personality Control."

34. Irving L. Janis, "Psychological Effects of Warnings," in *Man and Society in Disaster,* ed. by G.W. Baker and D.W. Chapman (New York: Basic Books, 1962), 55–92.

35. C. Fritz and E. Marks, "The NORC Studies of Human Behavior in Disaster," *Journal of Social Issues* 10 (1954): 26–41.

36. Ibid.

37. J.W. Powell, "A Poison Liquor Episode in Atlanta, Georgia," (Presented to the Conference on Field Studies on Reactions to Disasters, National Opinion Research Center, Chicago, 1953).

38. E.R. Danzig et al., "The Effects of Threatening Rumor on a Disaster Stricken Community," Disaster Study #10 (Washington, D.C.: National Academy of Sciences—National Research Council, 1958).

39. Janis, "Psychological Effects," 69.

40. Ibid., 70.

41. Fritz and Marks, "NORC Studies," 30.

42. Janis, "Psychological Effects, 57.

43. Dibner, "Ambiguity and Anxiety."

44. Vyner, "Psychological Effects of Radiation."

45. Ibid., 248.

46. Withey, "Reaction to Uncertain Threat," 118.

47. Frenkel-Brunswick, "Intolerance of Ambiguity."

48. B. Shalit, "Structural Ambiguity and Limits of Coping," *Journal of Human Stress* 3, no. 1 (1977): 32–45.

49. Lazarus, *Psychological Stress,* 117.

50. Susan Folkman, "Personal Control and Stress and Coping Processes: A Theoretical Analysis," *Journal of Personality and Social Psychology* 46, no. 4 (1984): 839–852.

51. M.E.P. Seligman, *Helplessness: On Depression, Development and Death* (San Francisco: W.H. Freeman, 1975); M.E.P. Seligman and S.F. Maier, "Failure to Escape Traumatic Shock," *Journal of Experimental Psychology* 74 (1967): 1–9.

52. J. Geer et al., "Reduction of Stress in Humans Through Non-Veridical Perceived Control of Aversive Stimulation," *Journal of Personality and Social Psychology* 16 (1971): 731–38.

53. H. Weiner, "The Concept of Stress in the Light of Studies on Disasters, Unemployment and Loss: A Critical Analysis," in *Stress in Health and Disease* ed. by M. R. Zales (New York: Brunner/Mazel, 1985), 84.

54. Shalit, "Structural Ambiguity," 34.

55. T.W. Milburn and K.H. Watman, *On the Nature of Threat* (New York: Brunner/Mazel, 1981), 31, 32.

Chapter 12

1. Irving L. Janis, "Psychological Effects of Warnings," in *Man and Society in Disaster,* ed. by G.W. Baker and D.W. Chapman (New York: Basic Books, 1962), 55–92.

2. Irving L. Janis and L. Mann, *Decision Making* (New York: The Free Press, 1977); Irving L. Janis, "Decisionmaking Under Stress," in *Handbook of Stress: Theoretical and Clinical For-Aspects,* ed. by L. Goldberger and S. Breznitz (New York: The Free Press, 1982).

3. Janis, "Decisionmaking Under Stress," 71.

4. Janis, "Psychological Effects of Warnings," 56.

5. Janis and Mann, *Decision Making,* 49.

6. Ibid., 11.

7. Ibid., 52.

8. Janis, "Decisionmaking Under Stress," 72.

9. Janis, "Psychological Effects of Warnings."

10. Janis and Mann, *Decision Making,* 59.

11. Janis, "Decisionmaking Under Stress," 77–78.

12. Ibid., 77.

13. Janis, "Psychological Effects of Warnings," 69.

14. Ibid.

15. Ibid., 71.

16. Ibid.

17. Ibid., 70.

18. Michael R. Reich, "Toxic Politics: A Comparative Study of Public and Private Responses to Chemical Disasters in the United States, Italy and Japan" (Ph.D. dissertation, Yale University, 1982), 26.

19. Adeline G. Levine, *Love Canal: Science, Politics and People* (Lexington, Mass.: Lexington Books, 1982), 110.

20. Ibid., 111.

21. Ibid; Martha R. Fowlkes and P.Y. Miller, "Love Canal: The Social Construction of Disaster" (Submitted to the Federal Emergency Management Agency, October 1982).

22. Henry M. Vyner, "The Psychological Effects of Ionizing Radiation," *Culture, Medicine and Psychiatry* 7 (1983): 241–63.

23. Janis and Mann, *Decision Making,* 78.

24. Janis, "Decisionmaking Under Stress," 73.

25. Janis and Mann, *Decision Making,* 78.

26. Ibid.

27. Ibid.

28. M.E.P. Seligman, *Helplessness: On Depression, Development and Death* (San Francisco: W.H. Freeman, 1975).

Chapter 13

1. J.M. Lopez-Pinero, *Historical Origins of the Concept of Neurosis* (Cambridge: Cambridge University Press, 1983), 14.

2. Ibid., 13.

3. F. Alexander and S. Selesnick, *The History of Psychiatry* (New York: Harper and Row, 1966).

4. Lopez-Pinero, *Neurosis,* 17.

5. Erwin Ackerknecht, *A Short History of Psychiatry* (New York: Hafner, 1968).

6. Henri Ellenberger, *The Discovery of the Unconscious* (New York: Basic Books, 1970), 46.

7. Ibid., 751.

8. S. Freud and J. Breuer, "On the Psychical Mechanism of Hysterical Phenomena: Preliminary Communication," Standard edition, 2 (London: Hogarth Press, 1955), 1–18.

9. Ellenberger, *Discovery of the Unconscious,* 758.

10. Mardi Horowitz, *The Stress Response Syndromes* (New York: Aronson, 1976).

11. S.S. Furst, "Psychic Trauma: A Survey," in *Psychic Trauma,* ed. by S.S. Furst (New York: Basic Books, 1967), 3–45; Phyllis Greenacre, "Infant Trauma and Genetic Patterns," in *Psychic Trauma,* ed. by S.S. Furst (New York: Basic Books, 1967), 108–53.

12. S. Freud, *Beyond the Pleasure Principle,* Standard edition, 18 (London: Hogarth Press, 1962).

13. K. Grinker and S. Spiegel, *Men Under Stress* (Philadelphia: Blakiston, 1945); Abram Kardiner, "The Traumatic Neuroses of War," *Psychosomatic Monographs II–III* (Washington, D.C.: National Research Council, 1941).

14. H. Krystal, *Massive Psychic Trauma* (New York: International Universities Press, 1968); P. Chodoff, "German Concentration Camp as Psychological Stress," *Archives of General Psychiatry* 22 (1970): 78–87.

15. Robert J. Lifton, *Death in Life* (New York: Random House, 1967).

16. A.W. Burgess and L. Holmstrom, "Rape Trauma Syndrome," *American Journal of Psychiatry* 10 (1974): 981–86.

17. E. Lindeman, "Symptomatology and Management of Acute Grief," *American Journal of Psychiatry* 131 (1944): 141–148; C.M. Parkes, "The First Year of Bereavement: A Longitudinal Study of Reaction of London Widows to the Death of Their Husbands," *Psychiatry* 33 (1970): 444–67.

18. M.R. Trimble, *Post-Traumatic Neurosis* (Chichester, England: Wiley, 1981).

19. Ibid.

20. American Psychiatric Association, Committee on Nomenclature and Statistics, *Diagnostic and Statistical Manual,* third edition (Washington, D.C.: American Psychiatric Association, 1981).

21. Kardiner, "Traumatic Neuroses."

22. Horowitz, *Stress Response Syndromes.*

23. S. Freud, *Introductory Lectures,* Standard edition, 15 (London: Hogarth Press, 1963), 273–86.

24. Kardiner, "Traumatic Neuroses," 82.

25. Ibid., 84.

26. Ibid., 82.

27. Ibid., 83.

28. Horowitz, *Stress Response Syndromes,* 94.

29. Ibid.

30. V.J. DeFazio, "Dynamic Perspectives on the Nature and Effects of Combat

Stress," in *Stress Disorders Among Vietnam Veterans,* ed. by C. Figley (New York: Brunner/Mazel, 1978), 23–42.

31. Freud, *Beyond the Pleasure Principle.*

32. C. Shatan, "The Grief of Soldiers: Vietnam Combat Veterans Self Help Movement," *American Journal of Orthopsychiatry* 43 (1973): 640–53; DeFazio, "Dynamic Perspectives,"

33. Lifton, *Death in Life.*

34. Burgess and Holmstrom, "Rape Trauma Syndrome."

35. Kardiner, "Traumatic Neuroses," 81.

36. Ibid., 116.

37. Ibid., 95.

38. S. Freud, "Inhibition, Symptoms and Anxiety," Standard edition (London: Hogarth Press, 1959), 80–86.

39. Furst, "Psychic Trauma," 37.

40. R. Janoff-Bulman and I.H. Frieze, "A Theoretical Perspective for Understanding Reactions to Victimization," *Journal of Social Issues* 39 (1983): 1–17.

41. Horowitz, *Stress Response Syndrome,* 22.

42. Furst, "Psychic Trauma," 28.

43. Ibid., 40.

44. Freud, *Beyond the Pleasure Principle.*

45. J. Sandler, "Trauma, Strain and Development," in *Psychic Trauma,* ed. by S.S. Furst (New York: Basic Books, 1967), 166.

46. Horowitz, *Stress Response Syndrome,* 20–21.

47. Henry M. Vyner, "The Psychological Effects of Ionizing Radiation," *Culture, Medicine and Psychiatry* 7 (1983): 241–63.

48. Adeline G. Levine, *Love Canal: Science, Politics and People* (Lexington, Mass.: Lexington Books, 1982).

49. Martha R. Fowlkes and P.Y. Miller, "Love Canal: The Social Construction of Disaster" (Submitted to the Federal Emergency Management Agency, October 1982).

50. Levine, *Love Canal;* Vyner, "Psychological Effects of Radiation."

51. Vyner, "Psychological Effects of Radiation."

52. Horowitz, *Stress Response Syndrome.*

53. Lifton, *Death in Life.*

54. C.M. Brodsky, "Psychological Factors Contributing to Somatoform Diseases Attributed to the Workplace," *Journal of Occupational Medicine* 25, no. 6 (1983): 459–64.

Chapter 14

1. U.S. Committee on Veterans Affairs, *Veterans Claims for Disabilities from Nuclear Weapons Testing* (Washington, D.C.: Government Printing Office, 1979).

2. National Research Council Committee on the Biological Effects of Ionizing Radiation, National Academy of Sciences, *The Effects on Populations of Exposure to Low Levels of Ionizing Radiation* (Washington, D.C.: National Academy Press, 1980); Interagency Task Force on the Health Effects of Ionizing Radiation, "Report of

the Interagency Task Force on the Health Effects of Ionizing Radiation" (Washington, D.C.: Department of Health Education and Welfare, 1979); United Nations Scientific Committee on the Effects of Atomic Radiation, *Ionizing Radiation: Levels and Effects* (New York: United Nations Publications, 1972).

    3. Abdel Omran et al., "Follow-Up Study of Patients Treated by X-Ray Epilation for Tinea Capitas: Psychiatric and Psychometric Evaluation," *American Journal of Public Health* 68, no. 6 (1978): 180–85; A. Peck and J. Boland, "Emotional Reactions to Radiation Therapy," *Cancer* 40 (1977): 180–85; L. Gottschalk et al., "Total and Half Body Irradiation: Effect on Cognitive and Emotional Processes," *Archives of General Psychiatry* 21, no. 5 (1959): 574–80.

    4. P.S. Houts et al., "Health Related Behavioral Impact of the Three Mile Island Nuclear Incident," Part III (Submitted to the Three Mile Island Advisory Panel on Health Research Studies of the Pennsylvania Department of Health, 1981); E. Bromet et al., *Mental Health of Residents Living Near the Three Mile Island Facility* (Pittsburgh: University of Pittsburgh Press, 1980); B. Dohrenwend et al., "Technical Staff Analysis Report on Behavioral Effects," (Presented to the President's Commission on the Accident at Three Mile Island, 1979).

    5. American Psychiatric Association, *Diagnostic and Statistical Manual, Mental Disorders,* edition two (Washington, D.C.: American Psychiatric Association, 1968).

    6. J.C. Nemiah, "Somatoform Disorders," in *Comprehensive Textbook of Psychiatry/III,* ed. by H.I. Kaplan et al. (Baltimore: Wilkins and Company, 1977), 924–42.

    7. E. Ackerknecht, "Paleopathology," in *Culture, Disease and Healing,* ed. by D. Landy (New York: MacMillan, 1977); G.M. Foster, "Disease Etiologies in Non-Western Medical Systems," *American Anthropologist* 78 (1976): 773–82; W.H.R. Rivers, *Medicine, Magic and Religion* (London: Kegan, Paul, Ltd., 1927).

    8. E. Ackerknecht, "Paleopathology."

    9. R.J. Lifton, *Death in Life* (New York: Random House, 1967), 119.

    10. Ibid.

    11. Field Research Corporation, *Public Opinion in Pennsylvania Toward the Accident at Three Mile Island and Its Aftermath* (San Francisco: Field Research Corporation, 1980); P. Houts et al., "Health Related Behavioral Impact"; E. Bromet et al., "Mental Health of Residents"; C.B. Flynn, "Three Mile Island Telephone Survey." (Submitted to the Nuclear Regulatory Commission, September 1979).

    12. Ibid.

    13. Ibid.

    14. Lifton, *Death in Life.*

    15. Field Research Corporation, *Public Opinion.*

Chapter 15

    1. Hans Selye, *Stress in Health and Disease* (Boston: Butterworths, 1976), 725.

    2. A. Baum et al., "Chronic and Acute Stress Associated With The Three Mile Island Accident and Decontamination" (Submitted to the Nuclear Regulatory Commission, July 1981).

3. C.M. Brodsky, "The Psychological Factors Contributing to Somatoform Diseases Attributed to the Workplace," *Journal of Occupational Medicine* 25, no. 6 (1983): 459–64.

Chapter 16

1. R.J. Lifton, *Death in Life* (New York: Random House, 1967).
2. H.M. Vyner, "The Psychological Effects of Ionizing Radiation," *Culture, Medicine and Psychiatry* 7 (1983): 241– 63.
3. C.M. Brodsky, "Psychological Factors Contributing to Somatoform Diseases Attributed to the Workplace," *Journal of Occupational Medicine* 25, no. 6 (1983): 459–64.
4. Field Research Corporation, *Public Opinion in Pennsylvania Toward the Accident at Three Mile Island and Its Aftermath* (San Francisco: Field Research Corporation, 1980).
5. Peter Houts et al., "Health Related Behavioral Impact of the Three Mile Island Incident," Parts I, II, III (Submitted to the Three Mile Island Advisory Panel on Health Research Studies of the Pennsylvania Department of Health, 1981).
6. H.M. Vyner, "The Psychosocial Effects of the Invisible Environmental Contaminants" (Presented at the Three Mile Island Public Health Fund's Workshop on the Psychosocial Effects of the Invisible Environmental Contaminants, June 1984).
7. H.M. Vyner, unpublished interview with an atomic veteran, July 1982.
8. Lifton, *Death in Life,* 121.
9. R.J. Lifton, *History and Human Survival* (New York: Random House, 1970), 168.
10. Lifton, *Death in Life,* 119.
11. Brodsky, "Somatoform Diseases."
12. Ibid., 460.
13. Ibid., 461–62.
14. M.R. Reich, "Toxic Politics: A Comparative Study of Public and Private Responses to Chemical Disasters in the United States, Italy and Japan" (Ph.D. dissertation, Yale University, 1982).
15. A.G. Levine, *Love Canal: Science, Politics and People* (Lexington, Mass.: Lexington Books, 1982).
16. M.R. Fowlkes and P.Y. Miller, "Love Canal: The Social Construction of Disaster" (Submitted to the Federal Emergency Management Agency, October 1983).
17. Irving L. Janis, "Decisionmaking under Stress," in *Handbook of Stress,* ed. by L. Goldberger and S. Breznitz (New York: The Free Press, 1982), 77–78.
18. Lifton, *Death in Life,* 105.
19. Vyner, "Ionizing Radiation"; H.M. Vyner, "Post-Exposure Health Care for Individuals Exposed to Radiation and the Other Invisible Environmental Contaminants," *Social Science and Medicine* (in press).
20. Reich, "Toxic Politics."
21. Brodsky, "Somatoform Diseases."
22. Lifton, *Death in Life,* 96.
23. Vyner, "Post-Exposure Health Care."

24. Ibid.
25. Reich, "Toxic Politics," 158.
26. Brodsky, "Somatoform Diseases," 459.
27. Lifton, *Death in Life.*
28. Fowlkes and Miller, "Love Canal."
29. Vyner, "Ionizing Radiation."
30. Lifton, *Death in Life.*
31. Brodsky, "Somatoform Diseases."
32. Fowlkes and Miller, "Love Canal."
33. Reich, "Toxic Politics."
34. Vyner, "Ionizing Radiation"; Vyner, "Post-Exposure Health Care."

Chapter 17

1. H. Wasserman and N. Solomon, *Killing Our Own* (New York: Dell, 1982).
2. J.L. Lyon et al., "Cancer Incidence in Mormons and Non-Mormons in Utah," *New England Journal of Medicine* 294, no. 3 (1976): 129–33.
3. A.G. Levine, *Love Canal: Science, Politics and People* (Lexington, Mass.: Lexington Books, 1982); M.R. Fowlkes and P.Y. Miller, "Love Canal: The Social Construction of Disaster" (Submitted to the Federal Emergency Management Agency, October 1982).
4. M.R. Reich, "Toxic Politics: A Comparative Study of Public and Private Responses to Chemical Disasters in the United States, Italy and Japan" (Ph.D. dissertation, Yale University, 1982).
5. Ibid.
6. Subcommittee on Medical Facilities and Benefits of the Committee of Veterans Affairs, House of Representatives, *Oversight Hearings to Receive Testimony on Agent Orange* (Washington, D.C.: Government Printing Office, 1981).
7. Wasserman and Solomon, *Killing Our Own.*
8. J. Hawkinson, *The Cyanide Controversy: A Toxicological Report on the Bhopal Gas Disaster* (San Francisco: Washington Research Institute, 1986).
9. D. Nelkin and M. Brown, *Workers at Risk* (Chicago: University of Chicago, 1984).
10. Wasserman and Solomon, *Killing Our Own.*
11. Subcommittee on Medical Facilities and Benefits of the Committee of Veterans Affairs, House of Representatives, *Oversight Hearings.*
12. Veterans Administration, *Claims Pursuant to Nuclear Test Participation* (Washington, D.C.: Government Printing Office, 1981).
13. Reich, "Toxic Politics."
14. Ibid., 307.
15. Ibid., 142.
16. M.R. Fowlkes and P.Y. Miller, "Toxic Waste at Love Canal: Experience and Perceptions," Unpublished manuscript, 109–10.
17. H.M. Vyner, "Post-Exposure Health Care for Patients Exposed to Radiation and the Other Invisible Environmental Contaminants," *Social Science and Medicine* (in press).

18. H.M. Vyner, unpublished interview, Israel Torres, March 1980.

19. H.M. Vyner, unpublished interviews, Andrew Hawkinson, February 1980.

20. H.M. Vyner, "The Psychological Effects of Ionizing Radiation," *Culture, Medicine and Psychiatry* 7 (1983): 241–63.

21. C.M. Brodsky, "Psychological Factors Contributing to Somatoform Diseases Attributed to the Workplace," *Journal of Occupational Medicine* 25, no. 6 (1983): 459–64.

Chapter 18

1. J. Pearson, "Hazard Visibility and Occupational Health Problem Solving: The Case of the Uranium Industry," *Journal of Community Health* 6 (1980): 136–47.

2. *UNSCEAR Report: Ionizing Radiation: Levels and Effects* (New York: United Nations Publications, 1972).

3. Pearson, "Hazard Visibility," 137.

4. Ibid., 138.

5. Ibid., 141.

6. M.R. Reich, "Toxic Politics: A Comparative Study of Public and Private Responses to Chemical Disasters in the United States, Italy and Japan" (Ph.D. dissertation, Yale University, 1982); M. Brown, "Setting Occupational Standards: The Vinyl Chloride Case," in *Controversy: The Politics of Technical Decisions,* ed. by Dorothy Nelkin (Beverly Hills: Sage Publications, 1979), 125–40; Adeline Levine, *Love Canal: Science, Politics and People* (Lexington, Mass.: Lexington Books, 1982); H.M. Vyner, "The Psychological Effects of Ionizing Radiation," *Culture, Medicine and Psychiatry* 7 (1983): 241–63; *Allen* v. *U.S.A.,* 588 F. Supp. 247 (D. Utah, 1984).

7. Vyner, "Ionizing Radiation"; Reich, "Toxic Politics."

8. J. Primack and F. von Hippel, *Advice and Dissent: Scientists in the Political Arena* (New York: Basic Books, 1974).

9. 588 F. Supp. 247, 211.

10. General Accounting Office, *Problems in Assessing the Cancer Risks of Low-Level Ionizing Radiation Exposure* (Washington, D.C.: General Accounting Office, 1981).

11. 588 F. Supp. 247, 233.

12. Ibid., 233–34.

13. Ibid., 246–47.

14. Ibid., 248.

15. Ibid., 269.

16. Ibid., 297–98.

17. Ibid., 289–90.

18. Ibid., 271–72.

19. Ibid., 252, 254.

20. Ibid., 270–71.

21. Reich, "Toxic Politics."

22. Ibid.

23. Ibid.

24. D. Nelkin and M. Brown, *Workers at Risk* (Chicago: University of Chicago Press, 1984).

25. Levine, *Love Canal.*

26. M.R. Fowlkes and P.Y. Miller, "Love Canal: The Social Construction of Disaster" (Submitted to the Federal Emergency Management Agency, October 1982); Levine, *Love Canal.*

27. 588 F. Supp. 247, 277.

28. Ibid.

29. Vyner, "Ionizing Radiation."

30. Levine, *Love Canal.*

31. Vyner, "Ionizing Radiation."

Chapter 19

1. Mary Douglas and A. Wildavsky, *Risk and Culture* (Berkeley: University of California Press, 1983).

Index

Acute radiation sickness: occasions of, 65–66; symptoms of, 65
Adaptational dilemmas, 30; definition of, 30; dimensions of, 18
Adaptational Model, 27–31, 99, 143–145; and precipitants of adaptation, 27–30; and uncertainty, 144
Ambiguity: as cause of stress, 88–91: in atomic veterans, 90; in carbon monoxide exposure, 89; in methyl alcohol contamination, 89–90; in psychiatric patients, 90; and hypervigilance, 96–98; as impediment to adaptation, 91–92; and mastery, 91; preservation of, 73
Ambiguity hypothesis, (Janis), 89
Anatomoclinical paradigm, 107
Atomic Bomb Casualty Commission, 15, 182–183, 185, 190
Atomic Energy Commission, 181, 183
Atomic veterans: case studies, 49–53, 125–127; diagnostic uncertainty, 50–51; etiological uncertainty, 51; history of, 121–122; identity conflicts, 129–131; medical mystery, 128, 133; operation crossroads, 49–50; patriotism, 130; post-test experience, 123–124; preoccupation, 128–129; radiation response syndrome (RRS), 121–140; self-diagnostic belief (SDB), 136; self-diagnostic belief system (SDBS), 133–137; undiagnosable symptoms, 50–51, 127; and Veterans Administration, 50, 52, 155

Benedikt, Moritz, 108
Bhopal, India, 168
Blaming the victim: atomic veterans and, 170–171; Love Canal and, 170; PCB and, 170; physicians and, 170–171; political conflict and, 167–168; psychological consequences of, 171–172
Boccacio, Giovanni, 11
Boundary uncertainty, 59
Brodsky, Caroll, 86–87, 152

Caffa, 5–6
Carbon monoxide asphyxiation, 96–97
Case studies: atomic veteran, 49–53, 125–127; Love Canal, 41–48; Michigan PBB exposure, 33–40
Charcot, Jean-Martin, 108–109
Cholera, 22–23
Clement VI, Pope, 11
Clinical pathology, 15–16
Cognitive appraisal: and mastery, 91–92
Cognitive theory: of stress, 67–73; of traumatic neuroses, 112–113
Coping behavior: and appraisal, 91–92; definition of, 72; functions of, 72; modes of, 72
Coping uncertainty, 63
Cullen, William: conception of central nervous system, 106; conception of the neuroses, 105

Delayed radiation illness: biology of, 15; non-tumorous forms of, 66; types of, 66

Acknowledgments

I would like to acknowledge the help of the following people and institutions:

Kaighn Smith, Jr.

Andy Hawkinson

Orville Kelley

Jim O'Connor

Tom Saffer

Susan Lambert

John Smitherman

Bob Alvarez

Kitty Tucker

Norman Solomon

Robert R. Holt

Robert J. Lifton

Lew Milford

Marty Teitl

Caro Pemberton

J. Truman

The CS Fund

Linda Lotz

Jim Hurst

Bob Coleman

Alida Rockefeller

Ann Roberts

Wade Green

The Kendall Foundation

Ruth Clark

Dan Hagan

The Three Mile Island Public
Health Fund

Pam Ferris

Adeline Levine

Neil Halfon

Dave Feigel

Mary Blackburn

Michael Muldavin

Elena Berliner

Dorian Kinder

Jim and Caren Quay

Marj Johntz

The Rockefeller Foundation

John Steiner

Jan Norman (Graphics)

Margaret Zusky

Marsha Finley

Nancy Herndon

Michael Attie

Cassandra Sagan

About the Author

Henry M. Vyner is a physician who has done six years of research on the psychological effects of ionizing radiation. The majority of this research has been done with military veterans who participated in atmospheric nuclear weapons tests and with the residents of the Three Mile Island area. Dr. Vyner received his M.D. from the University of Maryland and while a student held a National Institute of Mental Health Fellowship at Cane Hill Hospital in England. He has also been a Lowie Fellow in the Department of Anthropology at the University of California at Berkeley. His most recent position has been that of the director of research at the Radiation Research Institute in Berkeley.